A Compendium of

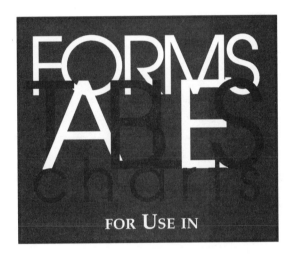

FORMS
TABLES
charts

for Use in

Monitoring and Evaluation

JOINT COMMISSION MISSION

The mission of the Joint Commission on Accreditation of Healthcare Organizations is to improve the quality of health care provided to the public. The Joint Commission develops standards of quality in collaboration with health professionals and others and stimulates health care organizations to meet or exceed the standards through accreditation and the teaching of quality improvement concepts.

Requests for permission to make copies of any part of this work should be mailed to:
Permissions Editor
Department of Publications
Joint Commission on Accreditation of Healthcare Organizations

ISBN: 0-86688-257-X

Library of Congress Catalog Number: 91-60207

Contents

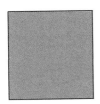

INTRODUCTION

The forms and related materials reproduced in this publication are intended to help you effectively carry out monitoring and evaluation of patient care quality. The nearly 180 forms, tables, and graphs are not presumed to be the "best" monitoring and evaluation forms ever created, but they are good ones. The selection is meant to be representative. Organizations may use them as examples upon which to base the design of their own forms. Before borrowing a form idea wholesale, however, each organization should make sure the form completely meets their requirements. In most cases the organization will want to customize a form to make it their own.

Table 1 lists the ten-step process of monitoring and evaluation.

Table 1. The Ten Steps of the Monitoring and Evaluation Process

1. Assign responsibility for monitoring and evaluation activities;

2. Delineate the scope of care and services;

3. Identify the most important aspects of care and service;

4. Identify indicators (and data sources, data-collection methods, and so on) for monitoring the important aspects of care and service;

5. Establish preliminary thresholds (levels, patterns, trends) for the indicators that trigger evaluation of the care and service;

6. Monitor the important aspects of care and service by collecting and organizing the data for each indicator;

7. Evaluate care and service when thresholds are reached in order to identify opportunities to improve care;

8. Take actions to improve care;

9. Assess the effectiveness of the actions and document the improvement in care; and

10. Communicate the results of the monitoring and evaluation process to relevant individuals, departments, or services and to the organizationwide quality assurance program.

Monitoring and evaluation is required throughout the clinical departments and services of all Joint Commission-accredited health care organizations (ie, hospitals, long term care organizations, psychiatric facilities, ambulatory care providers, and home care providers). This on-going process to assess and improve quality of care is a centerpiece in the accredited organization's quality assurance (QA) efforts. Monitoring and evaluation is a standard quality assessment and improvement process—simple, elegant, of proven effectiveness. The intent of the process is to help focus quality improvement activities on the most important elements of patient care and service through the collection and periodic evaluation of indicator data about key aspects of care and service.

This book includes examples of forms addressing each of the ten steps of monitoring and evaluation. (The word "form" is here used broadly for a variety of tables, forms, questionnaires, survey instruments, and graphs.) Of special interest are the forms used in systematically developing indicators (Figures 4.A through 4.E., page 31), and the data trending tables and graphs used in finding the cause of a variation in care and service patterns (Step 7, page 139).

The forms are, when practicable, organized by the step of monitoring and evaluation they address. Many of the forms may represent only a part or the kernel of what must be a larger form. Some are blank, others are filled out with sample information. Some of the forms are designed to be used in assessment and improvement activities within individual departments, others accross departments or organizationwide. In actual practice as in this book, it may be difficult or unnecessary for a particular health care organization to use a discrete form for each step of monitoring and evaluation.

This compendium also includes other types of quality assessment and improvement forms, notably

- forms used for the annual evaluation of a health care organization's QA program, and

- forms for displaying practitioner-specific information obtained through QA activities that are relevant to decisions about renewal/revision of clinical privileges or reappointment to the medical staff (and the appraisal of competence of individuals who do not have clinical privileges). (Practitioner-specific data lends confidence and objectivity to reappointment decisions; it is not gathered in order to punish practitioners. In those few instances where quality data identifies physicians in need of assistance, this information should be used in directing efforts to improve physician practice through educational efforts.)

As part of the chapter on evaluating care (Step 7), some of the main statistical and graphic tools used to continuously improve quality are illustrated in several places, especially Figures 7.W. and 7.HH. through 7.OO. (The procedures and philosophy of continuous quality improvement are discussed on page xii of this Introduction.) These tools are used to help staff understand and assess key hospital processes, focus improvement activities, and improve the processes. By 1994, Joint Commission standards will require an approach to assessing and improving quality based on the ideas and methods of continuous improvement. Monitoring and evaluation will continue to play an important role in these ideas and methods.

SOME CAVEATS

Essentially, these forms are ideas—hopefully good ideas—to help guide you in a particular step of the monitoring and evaluation process. The Joint Commission is neither requiring nor even officially "recommending" any of these forms.

For most of the steps of monitoring and evaluation process, *a form—of whatever type—is only one of many possible ways to carry out the step*; certainly any given form is not the only way to do a task. As stated in the scoring guidelines for Joint Commission medical staff standards, evidence of completing the steps of monitoring and evaluation may be found in *worksheets, meeting minutes, notes, memoranda, and QA plans*—not just forms. This compendium is not intended to encourage "papyromania," the compulsive accumulation of papers. In fact, probably the only step of monitoring and evaluation in which it is absolutely necessary to use forms is data collection (Step 6).

To cut down on unnecessary paper use, think about the *goal* of each step of monitoring and evaluation at the outset. This can cut down on the need for repetitive forms—for example, helping to avoid discussing one case through eight different medical staff committees.

Forms help document the monitoring and evaluation process, but each organization or department has to avoid being so structured that certain information is overlooked simply because it doesn't fit into a form or structure. Flexibility is important.

So is simplicity. "With adverse drug reaction forms, for example, the more information that staff has to fill in, the fewer adverse drug reactions get reported," says consultant Edgar Blount, MD, of Quality Healthcare Resources (QHR), Inc, a not-for-profit consulting subsidiary of the Joint Commission. "By contrast, one of the most effective drug reaction forms I've seen just had the definition of an adverse drug reaction, and the question 'Do you think this has occurred—yes or no?'—along with space for the staff member's name and the stamp of the patient. This simple form increased reporting of drug reactions threefold."[1]

One must balance the need for simplicity with the need for adequate information on forms, however. QHR consultant Shirley Noah, RN, recommends that more data than whether the indicator is met and the number of the patient in question be collected. It is hard to review the data in depth without initially collecting at least the number of the patient's practitioner and the shift, she explains.[2]

It should be noted that a few of the forms in this book contain "indicator" examples that are not well-defined indicators (eg, not objectively measurable). This compendium focuses on the forms that can be used, not the content of the samples.

Forms can prove helpful in facilitating monitoring and evaluation, but only if the goals and methods of the monitoring and evaluation process are well understood.

Perhaps by giving so many examples of forms we risk giving the impression that your monitoring and evaluation activities have to be very complex—after all, any process that could engender more than 170 forms must be complicated, right? In reality, however, most of these forms are creative variations on each other, giving you options on how to approach each step.

DATA ON LACK OF COMPLIANCE TO MONITORING AND EVALUATION

First introduced for Joint Commission survey in 1985 as the general paradigm for effectively and efficiently meeting the QA requirements, monitoring and evaluation standards have proved difficult for health care organizations to comply with ever since. As illustrated in Figure 1, page viii, 49 percent of hospitals surveyed during the 12 months ending June 30, 1990, received type I recommendations for "less than significant" compliance to standards for "Medical Staff/Departmental Monitoring and Evaluation." Other areas related to monitoring and evaluation (eg, Monitoring and Evaluation of Special Care Units and Radiology Services, Drug Usage Evaluation, Surgical Case Review) also accounted for a large percentage of hospitals receiving type I recommendations. (Essentially, a "type I recommendation" is a mandate, monitored by the Joint Commission, that an accredited health care organization improve its compliance with a given Joint Commission standard.)

Overall, Joint Commission standards involving monitoring and evaluation accounted for by far the highest level of type I recommendations in the 12-month period in question (although Safety Management and Life Safety were the single performance areas with the highest rates).

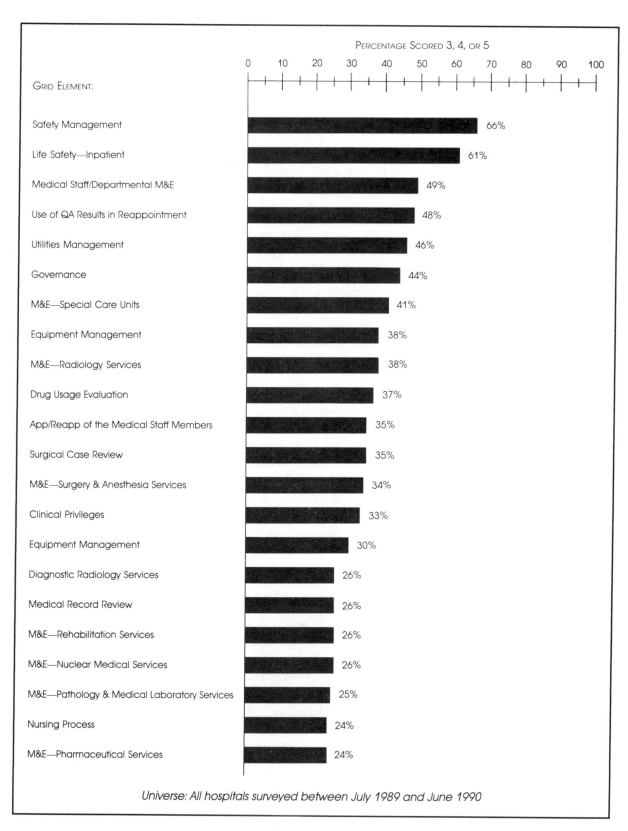

FIGURE 1. *Summary of Joint Commission grid element scores by percentage of hospitals receiving type 1 recommendations for "less than significant" compliance.*

This less-than-ideal performance is understandable since monitoring and evaluation requirements—like many Joint Commission standards—are meant to foster improvement, to stimulate hospitals to attain levels of performance beyond those needed historically. Compliance with these monitoring and evaluation requirements often requires a thorough restructuring of clinical management thinking and practice. Thus, a long learning curve is to be expected.

Type I recommendations are imposed when a hospital receives a survey score of 3 (partial compliance), 4 (minimal compliance), or 5 (noncompliance) on key requirements within any performance area listed in Figure 1. For example, the survey scores of those hospitals concerning Medical Staff/Department Monitoring and Evaluation break out as follows:

These facilities receive type I recommendations:

Substantial (Score 1) and Significant Compliance (Score 2)	Partial Compliance (Score 3)	Minimal Compliance (Score 4)	Noncompliance (Score 5)
51%	22%	24%	3%

(Hospitals that received type I recommendations in the performance areas listed in Figure 1 are expected to quickly improve in those areas. One or more focused surveys are scheduled for one to nine months later in order to check for improvement in compliance [and/or a written progress report must be submitted to the Joint Commission].)

Figure 2 is even more revealing. It shows the compliance rate of hospitals that received "conditional accreditation"—that is, demonstrated marginal compliance to Joint Commission standards—or that were denied accreditation. (About 6 percent of all surveyed hospitals received a conditional accreditation decision, and about 2 percent were denied accreditation because of poor compliance to standards during the year ending June 30, 1990.) Of these two groups of hospitals demonstrating the poorest compliance rates, a full 92 percent failed to achieve significant compliance to the standards for Medical Staff/Departmental Monitoring and Evaluation. Other Monitoring and Evaluation-related performance areas (Drug Usage Evaluation, Medical Record Review, Surgical Case Review, and Monitoring and Evaluation of Radiology Services) were poorly complied with by between 65 and 91 percent of this group of hospitals.

SPECIFIC DIFFICULTIES IN COMPLYING WITH MONITORING AND EVALUATION

What's the problem? Why are hospitals and other health care organizations having difficulty complying with the requirement for monitoring and evaluation? Experience shows the primary cause of type I recommendations to be Step 8, "taking action to improve care." In practice, health care organizations often get to the point of identifying a specific area where improvement is needed (eg, the source of a hitch in a system of care), but there is no evidence that they have done anything about it. In other cases, possible variations from a standard of care are labeled "approved" or "justified" by peer reviewers in almost every case, with or without a rationale. "Two kinds of inadequate 'action' which I see reported on QA reports are 'Will discuss the issue at next staff meeting' and 'Continuing to monitor same indicator,'" says Noah.[2] The reason these are not valid is that, in many cases, they are not designed to actually improve care. (Either, however, may be appropriate action in a *specific* case. It is seeing these as the *routine* action that is the problem.)

The challenge is how to initiate needed changes, which in many cases may involve more than continuing education. The forms included in this publication to address Step 8 may help focus the attention of QA committees on this concern.

What are some other difficulties health care organizations are having with monitoring and evaluation? Other areas that have caused poor compliance are

- not choosing measurable, well-defined indicators (Step 4, page 27).

- not choosing indicators related to the organization's important (high-risk, high-volume, or problem-prone) aspects of care (Step 3, page 23).

- not assessing the effectiveness of actions taken through continued monitoring and then documenting improvement (Step 9, page 209).

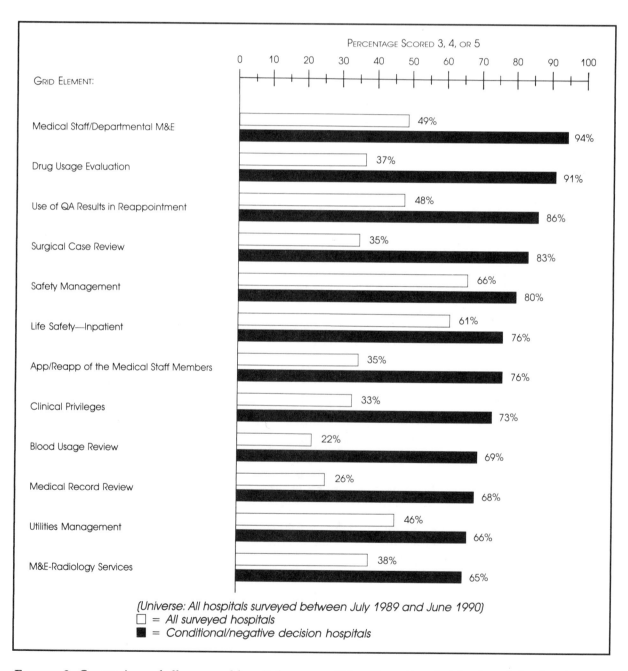

FIGURE 2. *Comparison of all surveyed hospitals vs. conditional/negative decision hospitals showing percentage that scored 3, 4, or 5 (ie, less then significant compliance) in Joint Commission type I performance areas.*

- lacking the time to do manual data collection, or lacking a sophisticated information system to aid in data collection and analysis.

- not understanding that when a given indicator reaches the threshold for evaluation, the process calls for the *evaluation* of patient care, not immediate action to improve care. When the threshold is passed many departments start looking to take action without first analyzing and discussing if there really *is* a need to change in order to bring improvement, according to Noah.[2] Without first understanding whether change is appropriate and then pinpointing what needs to be changed, it is unlikely that action taken will be on target. The best approach is first to do trend analysis (or, for a sentinel event such as anesthesia-related death, peer review) to understand what current performance is, then to pinpoint what must or can be improved, next to design an action to improve performance, and only then to implement the action. Looking at trends and patterns in data will help determine the scope of a possible problem, when and where it is happening, what needs to change, and what processes and who are involved.

- the person(s) with authority to approve recommended actions not reviewing and approving their implementation. Also, recommendations for action are sometimes not passed on to the specific individual(s) with the authority to approve them, or the person(s) is unaware of his/her responsibilities, or the recommendation is not specific enough to be acted upon even if it were approved. In other cases, the person(s) with authority doesn't evaluate and approve recommendation on a timely basis. Finally, if a recommendation is approved, the staff involved sometimes don't see it as an action they have to implement. There are many information/responsibility handoffs in which the "ball" can be fumbled, and often the main problem lies with a lack of commitment from top leadership to the quality improvement system.

- confusing thresholds for evaluation with standards of care. Not all thresholds need to be set at 0% or 100% so that every occurrence of the indicator requires an in-depth evaluation to see if improvement must occur. In the case of nosocomial infections, for instance, the medical literature tells us that even with the best of care, a certain percentage of patients get in-hospital infections. Therefore, setting the threshold above 0%, so that an evaluation is only *required* when the rate is above the threshold, may be an appropriate way to focus quality improvement activities on high-priority issues. The problem is partly that some hospitals are never willing to admit in public they do not have perfect care, says Noah.[2]

- trying to do too much monitoring and evaluation too soon. The Joint Commission scoring guidelines ask that at least two indicators be monitored in each hospital clinical department/service. This is a good level at which to start; hospitals can add to this number of indicators as they can handle more data, and make the called-for improvements.

- depending too much on sentinel events (ie, serious single occurrences such as maternal death), which call for peer review of individual cases, usually without improving systems of care and service. Concentration on sentinel events sometimes comes at the expense of looking at rate-based indicators that show trends of care and service and can lead to more significant changes in systems of delivery. Two problems with sentinel events are that (1) they are relatively rare, and (2) partly because of their rarity, they are not very good tools with which to teach how to rework and improve whole processes of care and service. In most organizations, concentrating on episodic sentinel occurrences does not predictably allow for adequate assessment of care and service to ensure that opportunities for improving care and service are identified and addressed. In any case, many sentinel events such as patient deaths are reviewed by the medical staff even without a monitoring and evaluation process. And

- failing to display and present data in a simple and persuasive format to the persons responsible for evaluating care and services and/or making changes. Step 7, page 139, addresses display formats.

Inevitably, a few difficulties in monitoring and evaluation compliance are also caused by or related to interpretation of Joint Commission standards language. As the QA standards have evolved, so has the monitoring and evaluation terminology, which—despite educational initiatives aimed at broadcasting the changes—still confuses some providers. Subtle changes of nuance in the Joint Commission's teaching of the ten-step process have also ocassionally confused some providers.

According to many sources, one contributing reason for lack of action taken to improve care and services has been the lack of involvement of physicians in quality assessment and improvement. This is supported by the data showing low hospital compliance with monitoring and evaluation-related activities (see Figure 1), indicating that physicians may not be fully engaged in traditional QA activities. Lack of physician involvement is especially serious because it is often the medical staff that must implement the actions that will improve clinical care and service (Step 8). Certainly there are several contributing causes for the lack of medical staff involvement—not least of which is the perception that QA is primarily focused on finding and punishing "bad" physicians rather than on improving poor systems of care, which are usually the source of problems.

CONTINUOUS QUALITY IMPROVEMENT

Good news for medical staffs is that the Joint Commission—and the health care field in general—is evolving from requirements for traditional QA (and its punitive associations) to fostering a continuous quality improvement approach (also called "total quality management," "hospitalwide quality improvement," or just "quality improvement" or "continuous improvement.") This shift will begin to be reflected in revisions in the 1992 Joint Commission QA standards, and will be fully reflected in the 1994 standards. Quality improvement emphasizes improving systems of care, rather than identifying outlier practitioners ("bad apples"). When diligently applied in industrial and service settings over a period of at least a half dozen years, continuous quality improvement enchanced quality, while also bringing cost savings and improving competitiveness; that is, it has demonstrated that improving quality does not cost *more*, it often costs *less*.

In brief, continuous quality improvement emphasizes

- a shift from the difficult task of "assuring" quality to trying to continually improve care.

- the belief that opportunities to improve are always present. "If it ain't broke, it can still be improved," is the motto of quality improvement, according to Dennis O'Leary, MD, the Joint Commission's president.[3]

- an organizationwide change in culture, so that everyone is involved in thinking about quality and improving processes of care, not just a single department that turns over quality reports. And

- the belief that most staff members are knowledgeable, competent, and want to do the best job they can, but are inhibited by the systems in which they work.

This shifts the emphasis from blaming doctors, nurses, or other staff members, to identifying how to improve the system. One reason physicians become enthusiastic about continuous quality improvement initiatives is that they've found what continuous quality improvement supporters predicted is true: "it's not 'worker' error, not incompetence, not malevolence that's responsible for most problems; it's a system, delivery, education or tracking problem," says Robert Klint, MD, CEO of SwedishAmerican Hospital, Rockford, Illinois.[4]

"For the average doctor, quality fails when systems fail: a test result lost, a specialist who cannot be reached, a missing requisition, a misinterpreted order, duplicate paperwork, a vanished on-call system," writes Donald Berwick, MD, associate professor of pediatrics, Harvard Medical School, Boston.[5] Thus, the physician who insists that his problems in caring for patients have been a result of the activities of the nursing staff, the governing board, and the decisions made by the administration will find that the quality improvement approach is providing a vehicle for those issues to be examined as part of the review of clinical care itself.

The quality improvement focus on processes and outcomes of care not only promises that care will be improved overall but also that staff will have a more positive attitude toward quality improvement methods since they are not placed in a defensive position.

For continuous quality improvement to work, "it is essential that the enormous talent, experience, and dedication already resident in the current quality assurance activities of our institutions be full integrated into our new quality strategies," writes Berwick. "What is noteworthy is not how irrelevant QA becomes in total quality management [ie, quality improvement] but rather how much its role expands."[6] Table 2 shows a terse comparison between traditional quality assurance (in this case, peer review as part of QA) and continuous quality improvement.

WHAT DOES THIS MEAN FOR THE ACCREDITATION PROCESS?

Monitoring and evaluation will continue to play a role in continuous improvement. Continuous quality improvement includes both (1) an organizationwide commitment to improving quality and (2) methods for the collection and use of objective data to assess and improve quality. Monitoring and evaluation both helps set priorities for assessment and improvement activities and provides some of the objective data for assessing and improving care and service. In the context of continuous improvement, it is an ongoing, comprehensive self-assessment system supporting and promoting continuous improvement in the quality of patient care and service. "What we learn from the success of quality improvement in industry is not that health care is doing too much measurement and monitoring, but that we're not doing

Table 2. Comparison of Peer Review and Quality Improvement

CHARACTERISTIC	PEER REVIEW	QUALITY IMPROVEMENT
Object of study	Physicians	Processes
Types of flaws studied	Special	Common and special
Goal	Control	Breakthrough
Performance referent	"Standard"	Capability/need
Source of knowledge	Peers	All
Review method	Summative	Analytic
Functions involved	Few	Many
Amount of activity	Some	Lots
Linkage of design, operations, and business plan	Loose	Tight
Tampering	Common	Rare

one zillionth of the measurement that we should," says Heather Palmer, MB, BCh, director, Center for Quality of Care Research and Education, Harvard School of Public Health, Boston.[7]

WHY FORMS?

What good does a form do? Forms are, of course, an organizing tool. They can make steps in a process explicit, thus allowing honest intellectual inquiry into how the process is set up. By showing the steps of logic in a process, forms help other individuals beside QA staff think through and understand the steps of quality improvement.

Forms are also a checklist to see if one has carried out every part of a process. They help people to be consistent, so that valid comparisons can be made between data and trends and patterns in data can be ascertained.

Making or filling out a form can also force one to plan—and to be realistic about plans—for example, to consider ahead of time in what manner and how often to do something like collecting data. And forms prompt people to do something. They can be a hedge against procrastination, by building in follow-up dates/loops.

An underlying purpose for forms such as those used for developing indicators (Step 4, page 27) is to get many people involved in setting direction. These forms can help get up-front agreement, understanding, and participation of everyone involved, so that later disagreements don't impede the process. Such forms can help prioritize.

It is true that forms used inappropriately or slavishly can in some cases limit creativity or put possibilities in a straitjacket. We hope you avoid that danger. The purpose of this compendium is not to limit your creativity or ideas, but rather to increase them.

REFERENCES

1. Personal communication between the author and E Blount, MD, consultant, Quality Healthcare Resources, Inc, a not-for-profit subsidiary of the Joint Commission, Oakbrook Terrace, Ill, Nov 1990.

2. Personal communication between the author and S Noah, consultant, Quality Healthcare Resources, Inc, a not-for-profit subsidiary of the Joint Commission, Oakbrook Terrace, Ill, Nov, 1990.

3. O'Leary D: President's column: CQI—A step beyond QA. *Perspectives* 10(2):3, March-April 1990.

4. Special report: Taking the fear out of quality assurance. *Medical Utilization Review* 8(9):6-8, May 10,1990.

5. Berwick DM: Continuous improvement as an ideal in health care. *N Engl J Med* 320(1):53-56, Jan 5, 1989.

6. Berwick DM: Peer review and quality management: Are they compatible? *QRB* 16(7):246-251, July 1990.

7. Personal communication between the author and H Palmer, MB, BCh, director, Center for Quality of Care Research and Education, Harvard School of Public Health, Boston, November 1990.

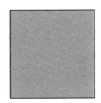 # OVERVIEW OF MONITORING AND EVALUATION

In Joint Commission-accredited organizations, the monitoring and evaluation process is a cornerstone of effective QA activities. The process is used by clinical services to monitor, evaluate, and improve care.

Ongoing medical staff monitoring and evaluation activities include departmental review, surgical case review, drug usage evaluation, blood usage review, and the pharmacy and therapeutics function. The process can also be used as part of *infection control, utilization review, risk management,* and *safety management.* Although each of these QA activities has its unique features and considerations, it is essential to understand the common framework of the monitoring and evaluation process.

Each chapter in this publication is divided into three main sections. First comes a description of one step of the process. Second comes notes on the place of forms in the step and specific points about the forms reprinted for that step in this publication. Third are the forms themselves.

The process for monitoring and evaluation is designed to help a health care organization effectively use its resources to improve the quality of care it provides. The individuals or groups responsible for various steps of monitoring and evaluation, the reporting processes, and the methods of integrating information will vary in different organizations. Of overriding importance is that

- monitoring and evaluation activities are ongoing, planned, systematic, and comprehensive;

- data collection and evaluation help to identify opportunities to improve care; and

- actions taken to improve care are effective.

The process by which care is monitored and evaluated can be understood by looking at the ten steps presented in synopsis form in Table 3, page 2.

Monitoring and evaluation is a "proactive" approach, intended to (1) identify those aspects of care and service that should be high-priority targets for assessment and improvement activities, and (2) identify which of those aspects of care or service must be the focus of immediate attention. Techniques such as monitoring and evaluation to quantify parameters of care and to systematically collect data also "allow individuals to 'externalize' a problem and look at it from a scientific point of view," write Paul Batalden, MD, and J. Paul O'Connor. "This approach is far less threatening than a more invasive and often emotional type of problem solving. Interestingly, people who 'think' they know what is wrong and believe the solution is obvious often are surprised to learn that their perceptions have been incorrect."*

Monitoring and evaluation is not only or primarily intended to identify *individual* cases in which care or service must be evaluated. Rather, the monitoring and evaluation process can be used to identify trends or patterns of care that may not be evident when only case-by-case review is performed. Whether focused on patterns or single events, the use of indicators helps to identify situations in which case review is necessary because it is most likely to identify opportunities to improve care and service. Although the monitoring and evaluation process will not identify every opportunity for improvement, it does help hospital staff identify situations on which their attention could be most productively focused.

Table 3. A Synopsis of the Ten-Step Monitoring and Evaluation Process

STEP 1: Assign Responsibility. The department/service should designate an individual or group (eg, medical director or QA committee) to be responsible for, and actively participate in, monitoring and evaluation. That individual or group assigns responsibility for the specific duties related to monitoring and evaluation.

STEP 2: Delineate Scope of Care and Service. Each department/service should establish an inventory of its activities. This delineated scope of care and service provides a basis for identifying those aspects of care and service that will be the focus of monitoring and evaluation.

STEP 3: Identify Important Aspects of Care and Service . Important aspects of care and service are those that are high-risk, high-volume, and/or problem-prone. Staff should identify important aspects of care and service to focus monitoring and evaluation on those activities with the greatest impact on quality and outcomes of patient care.

STEP 4: Identify Indicators. Indicators of quality should be identified for each important aspect of care and service. An indicator is a quantitative measure that can be used as a guide to monitor and evaluate the quality of important patient care and service activities.

STEP 5: Establish Thresholds for Evaluation. A threshold level, trend or pattern should be established at which indicator data will mandate that more extensive evaluation of the care and service must occur. For sentinel event indicators, the threshold is 0%. When such an event occurs, it must be evaluated.

STEP 6: Collect and Organize Data. Appropriate staff should collect data pertaining to the indicators. Data should be organized to facilitate comparison with the thresholds for evaluation.

STEP 7: Evaluate Care and Service. When the cumulative data related to an indicator reach the threshold for evaluation, appropriate staff members must evaluate the care provided to determine whether action to improve care should be taken. This evaluation should be sensitive to possible trends and patterns of performance. The evaluation should also attempt to identify causes of any problems or methods by which care or service may be improved.

STEP 8: Take Actions To Improve Care and Service. When opportunities to improve are identified, action plans must be developed, approved at appropriate levels, and enacted to improve care and service.

STEP 9: Assess the Actions and Document Improvement. The effectiveness of any actions taken should be assessed and documented. If further actions are necessary to improve care and service, they should be taken and their effectiveness assessed.

STEP 10: Communicate Relevant Information. Findings from and conclusions of monitoring and evaluation, as well as actions taken to improve care, should be documented and reported through the established channels of communication.

The Monitoring and Evaluation Process

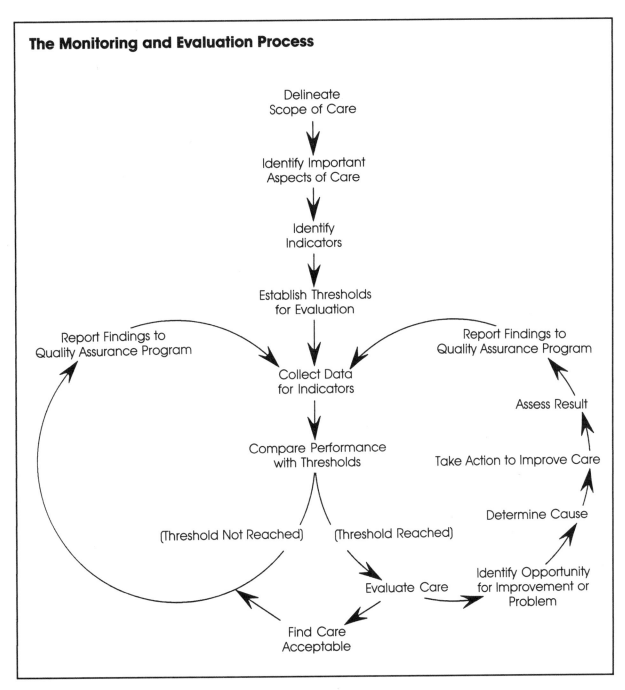

Figure 3. Visual representation of the monitoring and evaluation process as it functions from Steps 2 through 10. Appropriate staff members delineate scope of care, identify important aspects of care, identify indicators, and establish thresholds for evaluation to facilitate monitoring and evaluation of care provided in a particular department or service. Data pertaining to the indicators are collected, and the aggregate level of performance is compared with the threshold for evaluation. If the threshold is not reached, further evaluation is not necessary. Those findings are included in the regular report to the organizationwide quality assurance program. When the threshold is reached, the important aspect of care is evaluated to determine whether a problem or opportunity for improvement is present. If a problem or opportunity for improvement is identified, the cause is determined and action is taken. After a sufficient period of time, the effectiveness of the actions is assessed and the findings are reported to the organizationwide quality assurance program. Monitoring and evaluation is continued to identify any future deficiencies in care.

Although this book often approaches monitoring and evaluation as a department-specific process, the reader should remember that *inter*departmental assessment and improvement activities are often more effective than *intra*departmental activities, since so many of the processes that contribute to the quality of care and services are interdepartmental. For example, the process is used in cross-departmental activities such as drug usage evaluation, blood usage review, infection control, and so forth.

Without going too far afield to discuss the costs of monitoring and evaluation, it should be noted that a quality improvement program

- can use existing data sources to minimize paperwork;

- can be designed to use a minimum of staff time; and

- can result in significant improvements in quality and resource use if performed systematically and objectively.

Monitoring and evaluation in a continuous quality improvement era

The discussion that follows begins to look at steps of monitoring and evaluation in terms of how they can contribute to a continuous quality improvement approach. They are described here to help organizations to think about monitoring and evaluating care and services within a quality improvement context, not as requirements for compliance with current Joint Commission standards. As discussed in the Introduction, the monitoring and evaluation process will continue to play a role in the new standards that the Joint Commission will introduce over the next few years that are designed to foster continuous quality improvement.

The monitoring and evaluation process provides a solid point of departure for continuous improvement of quality. Setting priorities for assessment, developing methods and measures to monitor the priority aspects of care and service, objectively evaluating care and service, and taking actions to improve care and service are all part of in the current monitoring and evaluation process and will play a role in quality assessment and improvement in the future. In addition, however, some important expansions and modifications will be made as the Joint Commission revises its standards to foster continuous improvement in quality.

These expansions and modifications will include the following:

- Emphasizing the leadership role in improving quality;

- Expanding the scope of assessment and improvement activities beyond the strictly clinical to the interrelated governance, managerial, support, and clinical processes that affect patient outcomes;

- Utilizing other sources of feedback (in addition to ongoing monitoring) to trigger evaluation and improvement of care and services;

- Organizing the assessment and improvement activities around the flow of patient care and services, with special attention to how the "customer and supplier" relationships between departments (as well as within departments) can be improved, rather than compartmentalizing activities within departments and services;

- Focusing first on the processes of care and service rather than on the performance of individuals;

- Emphasizing continuous improvement rather than only solving identified problems; and

- Maintaining improvement over time.

In the 1992 *Accreditation Manual for Hospitals* the "Quality Assessment and Improvement" chapter will modify the 1991 "Quality Assurance" chapter and begin the shift toward continuous improvement of quality. The 1994 "Quality Assessment and Improvement" standards will be completely reorganized and revised, completing the shift.

Reference

*Batalden PB, O'Connor JP: *Quality Assurance in Ambulatory Care*. Germantown, MD: Aspen Systems Corp, 1980. p 12.

STEP

1 ASSIGN RESPONSIBILITY

Responsibility for seeing that monitoring and evaluation is implemented in a given department or facility is typically assigned to its chairperson or medical director (or a designee). In turn, this individual designates the responsibilities of other personnel in performing monitoring and evaluation activities (eg, identifying indicators, collecting data, evaluating care, and taking actions to improve care). The medical director also makes sure that those responsibilities are fulfilled.

Monitoring may also be cross-departmental. In that case the responsibility of departmental directors is to see that the scope of care in their departments are encompassed by the monitoring and evaluation activities.

Involvement of organizationwide leaders (eg, CEO, governing board and medical staff leaders, senior nursing leaders) is key to assuring an organizationwide commitment to quality improvement, to assuring that quality improvement is given high priority among the organization's activities, and that it includes those important processes that cross department/service lines. The leaders must also determine how they will help all staff learn the methods of quality improvement and foster staff's commitment to and involvement in the process.

Each department or service will, because of its unique characteristics and the structure of the particular organization it is part of, organize its monitoring and evaluation activities differently. These activities, however, should be performed as part of the staff's daily activities, use existing data sources when possible (to reduce paperwork and information-processing tasks), and include communication of QA goals and activities within and between departments and groups throughout the organization.

The following six forms simply show different frameworks for the assigning of responsibilities among staff and staff committees. Each form is a different way to show who is supposed to do what.

As mentioned in the Introduction, a form for this step is handy, but not absolutely necessary. The step could just as easily be performed by drafting a statement that clearly and simply describes responsibilities for each component of the process. Such a statement might begin as follows: ''In this department, the medical director is responsible for directing monitoring and evaluation activities; she will direct the delineation of the department's scope of care during a special meeting of all departmental staff. A team of three staff physicians and three nurses will make an initial proposal of important aspects of care for the medical director and staff to consider.''

Figures 1.D. and 1.E. are formats for showing who is responsible for monitoring and evaluation functions such as surgical case review, drug usage evaluation, medical record review, blood usage review, and the pharmacy and therapeutics function. For multihospital systems, Figure 1.F. shows a matrix that could be used to divide responsibility between hospital departments, single-hospital administration and governance, and various corporate headquarters management groups.

Monitoring and Evaluation Responsibilities

STEPS	Governing body	Medical staff executive committee	Physician director	Radiology quality assurance committee	Radiology administrator (nonphysician)	Radiologists	Technologists, nurses, and allied personnel	Clerical and/or medical record staff
1. Overall responsibility	✓	✓		✓				
2. Delineate scope of care				✓	✓	✓	✓	
3. Identify important aspects of care				✓	✓	✓	✓	
4. Identify indicators				✓	✓	✓	✓	
5. Establish thresholds				✓	✓	✓	✓	
6. Collect and organize data				✓	✓		✓	✓
7. Evaluate care				✓	✓	✓	✓	
8. Take action		✓	✓	✓	✓	✓	✓	✓
9. Assess actions				✓	✓	✓	✓	✓
10. Report relevant information			✓	✓	✓			

Comments:

FIGURE 1.A. Framework for the assignment of responsibilities for the monitoring and evaluation process among radiology department staff. A possible variation would be to make each box bigger and contain written details about that staff member's responsibility for the indicated step.

Monitoring and Evaluation Responsibilities Checklist

Activity	Responsible Individual or Group	Department Staff (Y/N)
Overall responsibility		
Designing monitoring and evaluation		
Delineating scope of care or service		
Identifying important aspects of care or service		
Identifying indicators		
Establishing thresholds for evaluation		
Establishing data analysis frequency		
Performing monitoring and evaluation		
Collecting data		
Organizing data		
Comparing cumulative data with thresholds		
Evaluating care when thresholds are reached*		
Taking action to correct problems		
Assessing effectiveness of actions		
Reporting conclusions, recommendations, actions, and results of actions to appropriate individuals or groups		

Evaluation may be divided into two phases—initial evaluation and more intensive evaluation when necessary.

FIGURE 1.B. *This checklist can be used to indicate the individual or group responsible for specific monitoring and evaluation activities and whether that party is within the department (eg, the chairperson, a department quality assurance committee) or outside the department (eg, quality assurance coordinator, medical records personnel).*

Assignment of Responsibilities for Monitoring and Evaluation

Department _____

1. Staff member/committee _____
Monitoring and evaluation responsibilities:

_____

_____

_____

2. Staff member/committee _____
Monitoring and evaluation responsibilities:

_____

_____

_____

3. Staff member/committee _____
Monitoring and evaluation responsibilities:

_____

_____

_____

4. Staff member/committee _____
Monitoring and evaluation responsibilities:

_____

_____

_____

5. Staff member/committee _____
Monitoring and evaluation responsibilities:

_____

_____

_____

6. Staff member/committee _____
Monitoring and evaluation responsibilities:

_____

_____

_____

7. Staff member/committee _____
Monitoring and evaluation responsibilities:

_____

_____

_____

FIGURE 1.C. *Example of a table showing assignment of responsibilities for monitoring and evaluation.*

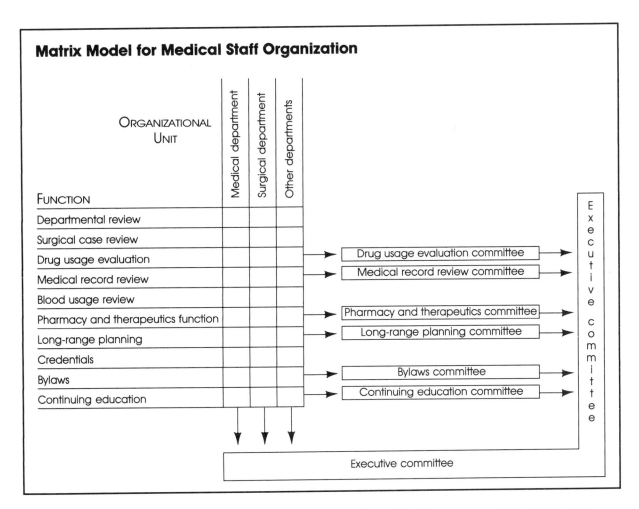

FIGURE 1.D. *Matrix model of medical staff organization illustrating the many possible relationships among departments and committees to accomplish the medical staff's QA responsibilities. Departmental involvement in a specific activity can be indicated by marking the appropriate box. In this example, the organizationwide medical staff has a committee to coordinate drug usage evaluation; individual departments report information on drug use to this committee, which in turn reports relevant information to the executive committee. The organizationwide medical staff in this example has no committee responsible for departmental review. Therefore, individual departments report their departmental review activities to the executive committee.*

Specific Departmental Responsibilities Matrix

DEPARTMENT: _____   ACTIVITIES: MONITORING AND EVALUATION

ACTIVITY RESPONSIBILITIES	Departmental review	Surgical case review	Drug usage evaluation	Medical record review	Blood usage review	Pharmacy and therapeutics function
Overall responsibility						
Delineate scope of care						
Identify important aspects of care						
Identify indicators						
Establish thresholds						
Collect and organize data						
Evaluate care						
Take action						
Assess actions						
Report relevant information						

Comments:

FIGURE 1.E. This matrix can be used to illustrate specific departmental responsibilities for monitoring and evaluation activities. Such a matrix can be used to support the organizational model shown in Figure 1.D., by clarifying areas of responsibility for the various medical staff activities. For example, a pediatrics department may have all ten listed responsibilities for departmental review, but may only assist in identifying indicators and establishing thresholds for medical record review.

Matrix of Responsibilities

PARTICIPANTS	INDICATORS AND STANDARDS		DATA ACQUISITION AND STORAGE		EVALUATION		STRATEGIES & INTERVENTIONS FOR IMPROVEMENT		REPORTS TO
	DIVISION SPECIFIC	CORPORATE-WIDE	DIVISION SPECIFIC	CORPORATE-WIDE	DIVISION SPECIFIC	CORPORATE-WIDE	DIVISION SPECIFIC	CORPORATE-WIDE	
DIVISION DEPARTMENT/ SERVICE	Develops and approves	Provides consultation	Responsible for data acquisition	Responsible for data acquisition	Prepares evaluation of dept/service specific data and indicators	Prepares evaluation of corporatewide data and indicators as appropriate to dept/sys	Develops, implements, & determines effectiveness as appropriate	Develops, implements, & determines effectiveness as appropriate	Division management—CEO and Medical Staff Executive Committee
DIVISION ADMINISTRATION & MEDICAL STAFF	Accountable for development	Accountable for consultation	Accountable for acquisition and storage	Accountable for acquisition and storage	Accountable for completing evaluations	Accountable for completing evaluations appropriate to division	Accountable for implementation	Accountable for implementation	Division Board of Trustees
DIVISION GOVERNANCE	Receives for information and comment	Receives for information and comment	Not applicable	Not applicable	Receives and reviews	Receives as appropriate to division	Receives for information as appropriate	Receives for information as appropriate	SMHC Board of Trustees
CORPORATE STAFF	Provides consultation and monitors development	Facilitates development	Provides consultation	Facilitates	Provides consultation	Prepares preliminary evaluation	Provides consultation	Provides consultation and reviews for effectiveness	Corporate Management
CORPORATE COMMITTEES & COUNCILS	Not applicable	Review and recommend	Not applicable	Review protocol for reliability & validity of data	Not applicable	Evaluate data	Not applicable	Recommend to corporate management	Corporate line management (Pres/ EVPs) through VP Prof Sys
CORPORATE MANAGEMENT	Accountable for development and approval	Accountable for development	Accountable for acquisition and storage	Accountable for acquisition and storage	Accountable for completing evaluation	Accountable for completing evaluation	Accountable for implementation	Accountable for implementation	SMHC Board & President of MHS
SMHC GOVERNANCE	Reviews as part of strategic planning process	Reviews as part of strategic planning process	Not applicable	Not applicable	Not applicable	Receives and reviews	Receives information as appropriate	Receives information as appropriate	MHS Board of Directors

FIGURE 1.F. Matrix of quality assurance responsibilities for a multihospital system. The matrix shows how to divide up responsibility for division-specific and corporatewide (systemwide) monitoring and evaluation steps. A similar form could be developed to divide chores between hospital departments, single-hospital administration and governance, and various systemwide corporate management groups.
SOURCE: *Sicher CM, et al: Sisters of Mercy Health Corporation Framework for Managing Quality. Farmington Hills, MI: Sisters of Mercy Health Corporation, 1987, p 20.*

STEP 2 ▪ DELINEATE SCOPE OF CARE AND SERVICE

One method to delineate the scope of care for a department is for staff to simply ask, "What is done in the department?" In answering this question, it is useful to review

- basic types of care and service provided (eg, inpatient, mental health);
- types of patients served (eg, age/sex/disability groups);
- conditions and diagnoses treated;
- treatments or procedures performed;
- preventive services provided;
- types of practitioners providing care and service;
- sites where care is provided; and
- times when it is provided.

The resultant inventory of activities provides a basis for subsequent steps in the monitoring and evaluation process; it helps ensure that all aspects of the care and service provided are considered when choosing those that are to be monitored and evaluated because of their degree of importance (see Step 3).

Another method of delineating the scope of care and service is to identify the department or organization's key governance, managerial, clinical, and support functions. All departments and services should contribute to this delineation of key functions.

Key functions are those functions that most affect the quality of care the patient ultimately receives, including clinical, support, managerial, and governance activities. Such key functions could include, among many others,

- medication use;
- blood use;
- nursing;
- infection control;
- diagnostic imaging;
- information management; and
- governance.

(A focus on key functions is not required by the Joint Commission. As of 1994, however, the standards in the *Accreditation Manual for Hospitals* will be organized around key functions, which should be among those the hospital addresses in its quality improvement activities.)

If the organization chooses this second method of delineating its scope of care and service, then the focus on quality improvement will be on understanding and improving these key functions.

One relatively painless way to come up with your scope of care and service is to gather patient care staff, and ask them the questions listed in Figure 2.A. As they offer responses, write them down on a flip chart; in 15 minutes you'll probably have completed the scope of care and service. Remember, the essence of this step is to simply write down the answer to the question "What do we do here (to and for the patient)?" This step should be relatively quick and easy, but thorough.

Figures 2.A. and 2.B. are forms used to help delineate your department's scope of care and service. The subsequent forms could be seen as special purpose forms or parts of larger forms. Figure 2.C. provides a structure to show scope of care and service for each department within a rehabilitation center. Figure 2.D. divides scope of care and service into aspects of care related to process and and those related to outcome, and by single disciplinary and multidisciplinary aspects of care.

Form to Delineate Scope of Care

DEPARTMENT/SERVICE _____

1. What are the significant activities and processes performed exclusively by the department/ service and what is the annual volume of each?

2. What are the diagnostic and therapeutic modalities used?

3. Who are the critical internal and external customers?

4. What types of patients are treated (eg, total number, demographic groups, inpatient-to-outpatient ratio, functional capability status, conditions and diagnoses represented)?

5. How does the department cooperate with, consult, and depend upon other departments, organizations, and professionals?

6. Who provides/performs the care/service (position titles)?

7. What/where are the sites of care/service (centralized, decentralized satellite)?

8. When are services provided (daily, weekly, monthly; shifts/weekends, and so on)?

FIGURE 2.A. *A form to help staff delineate a particular department's scope of care and service. Note that the first question asks for the number or volume of procedures performed annually; noting and listing such statistics can be a part of both delineating scope of care and service and choosing important aspects of care and service (Step 3).*
SOURCE: *Adapted from Evangelical Health Systems, Oak Brook, IL. Used with permission.*

Dept/Unit: ICU/CCU	Policy [X] Procedure [ ]
Final Administrative Approval/Date:	Department Approval/Date:
Medical Staff Approval/Date: Consultants/Date:	Committee(s):
	Source: Critical Care

New [ ]   Revision [X]   Date: 11/88

Scope of Care for the ICU/CCU—Policy Statement

PROCEDURES PERFORMED:

1. Continuous 24-hour EKG monitoring for all patients
2. Invasive hemodynamic monitoring with arterial lines, Swan-Ganz catheters, intra-aortic balloon pumps, intracranial pressure monitors, central venous pressure monitors, and temporary pacemaker
3. Initiation and/or maintenance of mechanical ventilatory assistance
4. Cardioversion—defibrillation technique
5. Initiation and/or maintenance of emergency and life support medications
6. Recognition and treatment of dysrhythmias
7. Assisting physicians with invasive bedside procedures

MEDICATIONS FREQUENTLY USED:

   All emergency medications per ACLS guidelines—vasopressors, vasodilators, antiarrhythmics, antianginals, narcotics, sedatives, volume expanders, blood products, diuretics, and parenteral nutrients

SERVICES PROVIDED:

1. Initial emergency treatment to stabilize patient with assistance from health care team
2. Managing medically chronic patients with cohesive care including psychological, emotional, medical, nutritional, and environmental needs
3. Providing partial or complete assistance with activities of daily living
4. Enlisting social service support for patients and families

TYPES OF PATIENTS—MAJOR CATEGORIES

Medical/Coronary Care

1. Coronary artery disease
   Myocardial infarction
   Unstable angina
   Cardiogenic shock
2. CVA
3. Drug or other substance, overdoses
4. GI Bleed
5. Multisystem organ failure
6. Cardiac and/or respiratory arrest
7. AIDS—with acute exacerbation of illness
8. Acute exacerbation of chronic obstructive pulmonary disease, pulmonary edema, congestive heart failure, or pneumonia

(continued)

Scope of Care for the ICU/CCU—Policy Statement (continued)

Surgical/Open Heart/Neurosurgical

1. Open heart surgery
2. Neurosurgery, neuro-trauma, and neurological infectious diseases
3. Multiple trauma
4. Postop, at risk, vascular, thoracic, and abdominal surgery

Other Aspects of Care

1. Management and Nursing care of critical patients with hemodynamic monitoring (ie, CVP/A-lines/IABP/ICP, Swan-Ganz) according to standards set by AACN
2. Management and nursing evaluation of monitoring of hydration and nutritional status of critical patients in collaboration with Nutritional Support Team
3. Planning, implementing, and evaluating the activity regime for critically ill patients
4. Management and nursing care of patients requiring ventilatory support in collaboration with Respiratory Therapy Dept
5. Management and nursing care of life-threatening arrhythmias according to ACLS protocol to include the prevention of
6. Prevention of nosocomial infection as reflected by IC Nursing statistics
7. Evaluation of rest and comfort of "critically ill patient" or "dying patient" as reflected by pain management incidence of ICU psychosis, patient satisfaction, and nurses' observation and documentation
8. Patient safety in regards to general environment equipment safety, structural safety as reflected by occurrence reports, surveys and biomedical reports
9. Client satisfaction (patient, employee, physician) as reflected by questionnaires, complaints, patient relations
10. Risk Management, problem focuses, or any concerns
    Quality care concerns will be reviewed by appropriate committees and individuals.
11. Unplanned admissions and appropriateness of admissions are reviewed
12. Annual privilege delineation for physicians and annual renewal of nurse qualification to assure competency in skills

Processes of Care

1. Accurate, detailed head-to-toe assessment on admission and every shift, with ability to readily detect any changes from the initial shift assessment. This assessment must be ongoing.
2. Ability to function in an emergency situation during Blue Alert and/or impending deterioration of patient condition. All staff certified in cardioversion and defibrillation.
3. Thorough planning of patient care and goal for each shift, with ability to reevaluate plan as necessary when an acute, unanticipated event occurs.
4. Act as resources to patients and their families regarding the hospital environment.
5. Patient education regarding health risk factors, knowledge of condition, and explanation of equipment used in ICU/CCU.
6. Conferring with physicians and other related health professionals in care of patient.
7. Communication between charge nurse and ICU physician regarding patient status while in ICU/CCU.
8. Preparation and planning with patient and their families/significant others to reach ultimate goal of transfer from ICU/CCU.
9. Provision of qualified nursing personnel with knowledge base sufficient to define patient's clinical status and potential problems; and to prevent, identify, evaluate, and resolve the abnormality in collaboration with health care team.

FIGURE 2.B. *A completed form showing the scope of care within a hospital intensive care unit.*
SOURCE: Memorial Hospital, Hollywood, FL. Used with permission.

Scope of Care for Rehabilitation Services

Department	Physical Therapy	Occupational Therapy	Psychological Services	Recreational Therapy	Rehabilitation Medicine

Major Clinical Functions	Physical therapy evaluation
	
	Physical therapy assessment
	
	Therapeutic interventions
	
	Application of modalities
	
	Patient and family education
		Assessment of occupational performance
		
		Treatment of occupational performance
		
		Therapeutic interventions, adaptations, and/or preventions
		
		Individualized evaluations and testing
		
		Patient and family education
			Assessment
			  Psychological
			  Vocational
			  Neuropsychological
			
			Interventions
			  Individual
			  Group
			  Family
				Assessment
				
				Treatment
				
				Leisure education
					Assessment
					Examination
					Medical management
					  Rehabilitation care
					  Medical conditions
					Coordinating individual rehabilitation program

Department	Rehabilitation Nursing	Social Work Services	Speech/Audiology	Vocational Rehabilitation	Prosthetics/Orthotics

Major Clinical Functions	Assessment
	
	Planning
	
	Intervention
	
	Evaluation
	
	Education
		Assessment of coping history, psychosocial adaptation to disability, family and support networks, and living arrangements
		Intervention to strengthen these behaviors and arrangements and to facilitate continuity of care
		Discharge planning
		Community service linkage/referrals
			Prevention
			
			Identification
			
			Diagnosis
			
			Consultation
			
			Treatment
				Assessment and evaluation
				  Testing
				  Counseling
				Results interpretation
				Recommendation
					Examinations
					Recommending prescription for equipment
					Designing and fitting
					Fit and function follow-up

Figure 2.C. Format to list major clinical functions in each department in a rehabilitation facility or unit. (Major clinical functions are key aspects of the scope of care; a similar form could be used to list a more complete scope of care for each department.)
Source: *Gray CS: Quality assurance in a rehabilitation facility: A decentralized approach. QRB 14(1):10, Jan 1988.*

Single and Multidisciplinary Aspects of Care

Scope of Care	Psychosocial well-being	Overall patient functioning	Primary medical care	Therapeutics
Single disciplinary aspects of care Process	Provision of appropriate single discipline programs (stimulation, entertainment, counseling, and so forth)	Assessments and treatment plans (activities of daily living, home safety, occupational therapy/physical therapy assessment)	Individual assessments (by physician, nurse, dietitian, and so forth) Appropriate response to emergencies	Individual assessments and treatment plans (structure: available supplies/space) Provision of special events
Outcome	Assessment of the effects of the single discipline programs	Assessment of the effects of single discipline interventions	Evaluation of treatment outcomes Timely diagnosis of medical problems Provision of appropriate medications	Evaluation of treatment outcomes Monitoring of patient attendance and meaningful participation
Multidisciplinary aspects of care Process	Development of appropriate treatment plans	Coordination of treatment plans	Management of appropriate responses from all disciplines regarding patients' medical needs Timely and appropriate testing	Coordination of disciplines to facilitate therapeutic programs
Outcome	Maintenance of patient motivation and peer group interaction Assessment of patient/family satisfaction Improvement of patient attitude and mood	Maintenance of patient condition, coordination, and ambulation Management of patient safety	Maintenance of overall patient functioning Keep patient in community setting	Improvement and/or maintenance of patients' functional level

Figure 2.D. *Form groups aspects of care by whether they are related to processes or outcomes of care, and by whether each is a single disciplinary or multidisciplinary aspect of care. This example is filled out by the staff of an adult day health care center.*
Source: *Richards HN, Hepburn K: Development of a quality assurance program in a medical model adult day health care center. QRB 15(3):84, March 1989.*

STEP 3 IDENTIFY IMPORTANT ASPECTS OF CARE

After the scope of patient care is delineated, staff members should ask themselves a more specific question: "Which of the things we do are most important to the quality of patient care?" The answer to this question should lead to identifying *important aspects of care*—the aspects on which monitoring and evaluation will be focused. To use the organization's QA resources (including professionals' time) as efficiently as possible, the activities, treatments, procedures, or key functions monitored should be those with the greatest impact (whether direct or indirect) on the patient outcomes. Therefore, priority should be given to those aspects of care and service for which one or more of the following is true:

- The aspect of care or service affects large numbers of patients (high-volume),

- The aspect of care or service is likely to affect the outcomes for individual patients if not performed, if not performed well, or if performed when not indicated (high-risk), and/or

- The aspect of care or service is suspected to be, or is considered likely to become, a source of problems (problem-prone). Indications of problems include controversy and disagreement over methods, technique, and efficacy; complaints on patient satisfaction surveys; suspected overuse or variability in use of resources; litigation from multiple cases involving the same specialty or diagnosis; and/or known or suspected high rates of complications or adverse results.

That is, high-volume, high-risk, and/or problem-prone aspects of care and service should be the highest priority for monitoring and evaluation. Organization resources and importance to the patient will also need to be considered when setting the priorities for important aspects of care.

Ultimately the number and scope of chosen aspects of care and service should reflect the full spectrum of care and service provided by the organization.

Following are three formats to support the process of identifying important aspects of care and service. Figure 3.B. shows how each important aspect of care and service can be rated by how many descriptors (eg, high risk, high cost, high volume) it fulfills. As indicated by Figure 3.C., choosing important aspects of care and service should be a data-driven process (eg, which procedures do staff do the most or have the most complications with).

C or S	IMPORTANT ASPECTS OF CARE/SERVICE	SE	SR	PP	SI

C = An aspect of care identified as a key customer-defined requirement
S = An aspect of care that may not be visible to your customer, but is important to the accomplishments of the unit because of its effect on suppliers/providers of care
SE = Significant effect on process/outcome of care
SR = Significant risk to patient
PP = Problem prone
SI = Significant impact on unit's role

FIGURE 3.A. *Form to determine important aspects of care and service. This form helps describe each aspect of care and service by whether it is important primarily to customers (receivers of the department's services) or suppliers (anyone who provides services to the department).*
SOURCE: *Adapted from Evangelical Health Systems, Oak Brook, IL. Used with permission.*

Drug Evaluation Matrix

DRUG	HIGH VOLUME	HIGH COST	HIGH RISK	PROBLEM PRONE	NARROW THERAPEUTIC RANGE	TOTAL
A	yes	yes	yes	yes	yes	5
B	no	yes	yes	yes	no	3
C	no	no	no	yes	yes	2

FIGURE 3.B. *This matrix shows how important aspects of care and service—in this case, particular drugs—can be rated by how many descriptors (eg, high risk, high cost, high volume) each fulfills. Such a matrix can be used to prioritize which important aspects of care and service to monitor.*
SOURCE: *Bunting RF: A model drug usage evaluation program.* Journal of Quality Assurance 12(3): 31, Jul/Aug 1990.

Worksheet for Determining Important Aspects of Care

DEPARTMENT _____ PERSON COMPLETING _____

List five most frequent procedures/services:
1. _____
2. _____
3. _____
4. _____
5. _____

List five most frequent diagnoses:

PROCEDURE	AVERAGE NUMBER PER MONTH
1. _____	_____
2. _____	_____
3. _____	_____
4. _____	_____
5. _____	_____

List services involving high risk to patients:
1. _____
2. _____
3. _____
4. _____
5. _____

List the four surgical procedures with the highest rates of intraoperative and postoperative complications:

PROCEDURE	AVERAGE MONTHLY COMPLICATION RATE
1. _____	_____
2. _____	_____
3. _____	_____
4. _____	_____
5. _____	_____

List the two types of incidents that your department reported most often to the risk management department in the last six months:
1. _____
2. _____

List new procedures performed, drugs, or major new equipment obtained in the last nine months:
1. _____
2. _____
3. _____
4. _____
5. _____

List infection control problems reported or identified in the last 12 months:
1. _____
2. _____
3. _____
4. _____
5. _____

(continued)

Worksheet for Determining Important Aspects of Care (continued)

List examples of the following:*

Unexplained variation in clinical practice   _____
_____
_____

Unexplained variation in utilization of   _____
limited or costly resources   _____

Unexplained variation in internal or   _____
external referral patterns   _____

General clinical uncertainty or controversy   _____
_____
_____

Uncertain indications for risky or costly   _____
intervention   _____

List quality-of-care problems perceived by   1. _____
patients, clinicians, or managers: 2. _____
3. _____
4. _____

---

*The following questions are adapted from Gottlieb LK, Margolis CZ, Schoenbaum SC: Clinical practice guidelines at an HMO: Development and implementation in a quality improvement model. QRB 16(2):81, Feb 1990.

FIGURE 3.C. *A worksheet such as this can help department staff identify the high-volume, high-risk, and/or problem-prone activities that should be monitored, by asking for particular information (eg, which procedures do staff do the most/have the most complications with).*

STEP 4 IDENTIFY INDICATORS

To efficiently evaluate the care and service provided, performance indicators should be identified. An indicator is *a quantitative measure that can be used as a guide to monitor and evaluate the quality of important patient care and support service activities.* The emphasis should be on indicators that measure activities that are important for patient outcomes, not, for example, merely medical record keeping.

Indicators are used to collect data about important aspects of care and service and to direct attention toward opportunities for improvement. They should be objective and reliable measures of the processes and/or outcomes of the important aspects of care.

Measures of processes include, for example, whether a specific diagnostic test was performed before medication was prescribed, the time between diagnosis and a required emergency intervention, and whether an appropriate indication was present for a specific surgical procedure. Process indicators for direct care processed may be based upon established practice guidelines or parameters. For example, if a practice guideline states that the serum level of a certain drug should be maintained within specific limits, an indicator of this important aspect of care might be how often the serum level falls outside those limits.

Measures of outcomes used as indicators might include the complication rate for a specific surgical procedure, the length of stay for treatment of a specific disease, the rate of adverse drug reactions, and the functional level of a rehabilitation patient. As these examples illustrate, outcome measures may range from the immediate outcome of a specific procedure (eg, a transfusion reaction) to an intermediate outcome related to a specific treatment (eg, development of a surgical wound infection after surgery) to a short-term outcome of hospital treatment (eg, length of stay for a specific illness) to a long-term outcome (eg, functional work status of a rehabilitation patient).

Occurrence(s) of an undesired outcome (eg, transfusion reaction) identified by an indicator does not necessarily indicate a problem in the quality of care. Evaluation is necessary to ascertain the cause of the outcome and whether changes should be made to improve the outcomes.

Indicators should clearly state exactly which discrete, concrete *data elements* must be collected. Take, for example, the following Joint Commission recommended obstetrics indicator:

> *Patients with excessive maternal blood loss defined by either postdelivery red blood cell transfusion or a low postdelivery hematocrit or hemoglobin (Hct 22%, Hgb 7 grams) or a significant predelivery to postdelivery decrease in hematocrit (decrease $\geq$ 11%) or hemoglobin (decrease $\geq$ 3.5 grams), excluding patients with abruptio placenta previa.*

This indicator specifies objective data elements to be recorded, such as specific hemoglobin and hematocrit levels and incidence of postdelivery red blood cell transfusion.

As feasible, indicators should be derived from authoritative sources and supported by the best available clinical and QA literature. Indicators should be selected, developed, and/or adapted by staff members who are expert in the clinical area. Those knowledgeable individuals that formulate indicators may be drawn from within one department or from a number of departments.

DATA SOURCES FOR EACH INDICATOR

Finally an indicator is made "operational" by not only describing which objective data are to be collected, but also where the data are to be found—in the medical record, in the case of the maternal blood loss indicator—and which staff members are to be involved in collecting the data.

The individual, groups, or teams who develop indicators and thresholds are in the best position to identify sources for data pertaining to each indicator. The source of data will vary depending on the indicator, but the following are some common places quality-related data can be found:

- patient records;
- laboratory reports;
- incident reports;
- medication logs;
- financial data;
- patient satisfaction questionnaires;
- autopsy reports;
- infection control reports;
- direct observation and measurement; and
- utilization review findings.

An indicator's data elements will govern the selection of data sources.

Once the data source is chosen, those who developed the indicators are also in a good position to help determine which data-collection methodology is appropriate.

DATA-COLLECTION METHOD

A data-collection methodology must be chosen and established. Designing and establishing this methodology entails deciding who will collect data and whether collection will be concurrent or retrospective.

Because data collection that follows the flow of patient care often crosses departmental lines and involves the entire organization, cross-departmental teams or individuals often oversee design of the data collection methods. To minimize the investment of organization resources, the most efficient data collection process should be established, one that takes into account data-collection already being carried out (eg, for utilization review purposes) in the organization.

In some cases, department members providing the care to be monitored perform the actual data collection. Department clerical staff may be able to collect data if the individuals are appropriately trained and if indicators are specific and well defined. In other cases, an individual or group from outside the department (such as medical records or quality assurance personnel) collects data. Increasing numbers of health care organizations have computer systems with which to collect and manage QA and other data.

The forms are presented in the following four groups:

1. Indicator Development Forms (Figures 4.A. through 4.E.). The Joint Commission's own form used in developing its Agenda for Change indicators (Figure 4.A.) is followed by the same form filled in for one of the Joint Commission recommended obstetrics indicators (Figure 4.B.). Figures 4.C. and 4.D. are two other examples of indicator development forms.

These are forms designed to guide staff members in systematically formulating new indicators. A form or worksheet used to help develop indicators can clarify every aspect of an indicator—eg, the patient population being monitored, which data elements are to be collected and when, why this indicator is an important measure, data source(s), data collector, and method of tabulating and evaluating the data. If all this is not agreed to by all appropriate staff members and made explicit (as a form can do) when the indicator is developed, staff may raise objections at the end of the process, once data have been collected and actions are being taken to improve care. If, in the process of filling out an indicator development form, practitioners are involved in choosing indicators, the practitioners will not be likely to miss the significance of the findings once the data is collected.

Indicator development forms help guide and document the process of developing indicators. Such a form should usually include at least the following elements:

- Initial statement of the indicator;
- Definition of terms (to assure that everyone is collecting and measuring the same data elements);
- Rationale (ie, evidence that a given indicator is in fact important or useful to measure);
- Data collection information (eg, how to collect data, source, optional source, data collector, sampling technique, frequency of collection); and
- Evaluation (eg, how data collection will be evaluated, how other factors such as severity of illness and comorbid conditions will affect the indicator data).

Two major goals of the indicator development process are (1) to choose indicators in a way that makes efficient and effective use of organization and expert resources, and (2) to achieve expert consensus on a set of clinically valid indicators.

Developing an indicator includes choosing the appropriate data sources and data-collection method to monitor the indicator. Figure 4.E. is a checklist to gauge the adequacy of the data collection tool and method.

Of course, any indicator developed with the help of a form such as those in Figures 4.A. through 4.E. still needs to be tested *in use* to see if, as written, it can be reliably collected and analyzed to provide feedback to providers, to assess its value in raising questions about patient care that help determine if care and services can be improved, and to assess the ability of the indicators to describe accurately the organization's performance.

2. Forms allowing multiple practitioners to rate proposed indicators (Figures 4.F. through 4.P.). By letting practitioners rate, comment upon, or vote on proposed indicators, these forms can help refine indicators, build staff consensus, and choose the best indicators from a group of alternatives.

Figure 4.F. is a rating form developed by the Joint Commission to get expert opinion on its proposed Agenda for Change indicators. It is a survey form given to practitioners to elicit their opinion of the clinical relevance of proposed indicators. At a later stage, shortly before field testing an indicator, the Joint Commission uses the survey form in Figure 4.G. to get expert opinion on the completeness and "data collectibility" of an indicator. Figures 4.H. and 4.I. are forms for a similar task. When field testing of new indicators has begun, questionnaires such as 4.J. and 4.K. can be used to gather staff members' perceptions and recommendations concerning the value of indicators and their ease of use. Figure 4.L. is a three-part mechanism practitioners can use to weight proposed indicators according to their priority and to revise those weights through a a modified Delphi process. Figure 4.M. shows elements of care for acute tonsillitis weighted by physicians for importance ("3.0" indicating the greatest importance); this sort of weighting may be done to help determine the most important elements of care to monitor. Figure 4.N. shows the results of panelists' ratings of the possible indications for carotid endarterectomy (which can become the basis of a performance-related indicator). Figures 4.O. and 4.P. can be used to help evaluate the appropriateness of indicators already in use and prioritize monitoring the important aspects of care that the indicators address.

3. Forms to list or describe indicators (Figures 4.Q. through 4.W.). (Some of these forms have been filled out with sample indicators.) Figure 4.Q. is the Joint Commission's form to list indicator data elements and definitions (in this case, for the indicator used as an example in Figure 4.B.) Figure 4.T. provides a format for identifying and analyzing suspected problems that may be assessed through development and application of indicators.

Figures 4.U. through 4.W. address an important aspect of preparing indicators for monitoring: the setting of data collection strategy.

4. Patient/Staff Satisfaction Surveys (Figures 4.X. through 4.LL.). Such survey questionnaires generate data that can reveal the need for indicator-based monitoring of various aspects of care and service. The questions in satisfaction surveys are themselves monitors of quality, and the survey sheet itself is a data collection tool. Included are

– a satisfaction survey questionnaire regarding hospital care (Figure 4.X.),
– a survey questionnaire for children (and their parents) cared for in a hospital (Figure 4.Y.),
– an ambulatory care center satisfaction survey questionnaire (Figure 4.Z.),
– an interview script for a patient satisfaction survey conducted by telephone (Figure 4.BB.),
– an instrument to measure patient satisfaction within a particular hospital department (Figure 4.CC.), and
– a food service satisfaction survey questionnaire (Figure 4.DD.).

Other forms are designed for recording a patient complaint, compiling a monthly summary report about patient problems/complaints, and recording the impressions of a "mystery visitor" hired by the hospital to visit the hospital and rate its service.

Also included are surveys to rate the satisfaction of staff members with internal services and with their jobs and work environment (Figures 4.JJ. through 4.LL.). Staff satisfaction with internal services is important; a particular hospital department's "customers" are not only patients but also other departments and staff members.

Clinical Indicator Development Form

I. INDICATOR
    A.

    B.

II. DEFINITION OF TERMS
    (Define terms contained in the indicator which may be ambiguous or need further explanation for collection purposes.)

III. TYPE OF INDICATOR
    A. Expected Level of Analysis
        Indicate the approach that would be expected of hospitals in response to this indicator.
        ☐ sentinel event indicator: all occurrences warrant review by the hospital.
        ☐ rate-based indicator: further assessment by the hospital is warranted if the occurrence rate shows a noticeable trend over time or indicates statistically significant differences when compared to peer institutions.

    B. This indicator primarily addresses
        ☐ a process of patient care.
        ☐ a patient outcome.

IV. RATIONALE
    A. Indicate the reason why this indicator is useful to assess and the specific patient process or outcome that will be monitored.

    B. Selected references (Identify the sources of information used to develop the above rationale.)

    C. Identify the practitioner and/or organizational processes assessed by this indicator and rate the importance of each.

	Somewhat Important	Important	Very Important	Essential*
1. _____	1	2	3	4
2. _____	1	2	3	4
3. _____	1	2	3	4
4. _____	1	2	3	4
5. _____	1	2	3	4

V. DESCRIPTION OF INDICATOR POPULATION
    A. Subcategories (Identify patient subpopulations by which the indicator data will be separated for analysis.)

    B. Data Format (Define the manner by which the population will be expressed.)
        1. Numerator(s):
        2. Denominator(s):

*This rating chart is optional.   (continued)

Clinical Indicator Development Form (continued)

VI.   REQUIRED DATA ELEMENTS AND LOGIC
List the specific data elements to be collected and the logic (eg, ICD-9-CM code) that will
identify the patients assessed by the indicator. Also, enter the most likely sources of
documentation (eg, anesthesia report) for each data element identified on the left.

Data Elements   *Data Sources*

A.   1. _____
                                                            2. _____
                                                            3. _____
B.   1. _____
                                                            2. _____
                                                            3. _____
C.   1. _____
                                                            2. _____
                                                            3. _____
D.   1. _____
                                                            2. _____
                                                            3. _____

VII.   UNDERLYING FACTORS
(List factors not included in the indicator that may account for significant indicator rates or
indicator activity. Reference and rate each factor in terms of its relative importance in
interpreting indicator data.)

A.   Patient-based factors (ie, factors outside the health care organization's control
contributing to patient outcomes)
1.   Severity of illness (ie, factors related to the degree or stage of disease prior to
treatment)

	Not Important				Very Important*
a. _____	1	2	3	4	5
b. _____	1	2	3	4	5
c. _____	1	2	3	4	5
d. _____	1	2	3	4	5
e. _____	1	2	3	4	5
f. _____	1	2	3	4	5

References: _____
_____
_____

2.   Comorbid conditions (ie, disease factors, not intrinsic to the primary disease, which
may have an impact on patient suitability for, or tolerance of, diagnostic or
therapeutic care)

	Not Important				Very Important*
a. _____	1	2	3	4	5
b. _____	1	2	3	4	5
c. _____	1	2	3	4	5
d. _____	1	2	3	4	5
e. _____	1	2	3	4	5
f. _____	1	2	3	4	5

*This rating chart is optional.

(continued)

Clinical Indicator Development Form (continued)

References: _____
_____
_____

3. Other patient factors (ie, nondisease factors that may have an impact on care—eg, age, sex, refusal of consent)

		Not Important				Very Important*
a. _____		1	2	3	4	5
b. _____		1	2	3	4	5
c. _____		1	2	3	4	5
d. _____		1	2	3	4	5
e. _____		1	2	3	4	5
f. _____		1	2	3	4	5

References: _____
_____
_____

4. Risk Adjustment Factors: Identify which of the above underlying causes should be collected as risk adjustment factors and the respective data elements that define the factors and sources of data.

Underlying factor	Data element	Source
a. _____	a. _____	a. _____
b. _____	b. _____	b. _____
c. _____	c. _____	c. _____

5. If any factors above (VII 4 a-c) should be used to define the indicator itself, and thereby added to the indicator statement, circle the appropriate factors above.

B. Non–patient-based factors (ie, factors within the health care organization's control or problem areas causing indicator activity)

		Not Important				Very Important*
a. _____		1	2	3	4	5
b. _____		1	2	3	4	5
c. _____		1	2	3	4	5
d. _____		1	2	3	4	5
e. _____		1	2	3	4	5
f. _____		1	2	3	4	5

References: _____
_____
_____

VIII. EXISTING DATA BASES:
Are there research or clinically operational data bases from which indicator occurrence rates and/or institutional variance could be established/verified?

This rating chart is optional.

FIGURE 4.A. *The Joint Commission's clinical indicator development form. A hospital or hospital system may use a form of this type to develop its own indicators in a systematic manner. The form helps ensure that each indicator developed is objective and measurable, specifying the source of data, and so on.*

Obstetrical Care Indicator Development Form

I. INDICATOR
   A. **OB-3. MATERNAL BLOOD LOSS**

   B. Patients with excessive maternal blood loss defined by intra and/or postpartum red blood cell transfusion or a low postdelivery hematocrit or hemoglobin (Hct < 22%, Hgb < 7 gms) or a significant pre- to postdelivery decrease in hematocrit ($\geq$ 11%) or hemoglobin ($\geq$ 3.5 gms) excluding patients with abruptio placenta or placenta previa.

II. DEFINITION OF TERMS
   Predelivery Hgb/Hct: the most recent Hgb or Hct value within 1 month prior to delivery.

   Postdelivery Hgb/Hct: the lowest value recorded subsequent to delivery and prior to hospital discharge.

   Transfusion includes:
      autotransfusion of whole blood (99.02)
      other transfusion of whole blood (99.03)
      transfusion of packed cells (99.04)

   Primary Exclusion Criteria:
      If maternal diagnosis:
      placenta previa without hemorrhage (641.01)
      hemorrhage from placenta previa (641.11)
      premature separation of placenta, abruptio (641.21)

III. TYPE OF INDICATOR
   A. Expected Level of Analysis
      ☐ sentinel event indicator: all occurrences warrant review by the hospital.

      ☒ rate-based indicator: further assessment by the hospital is warranted if the occurrence rate shows a noticeable trend over time or indicates statistically significant differences when compared to peer institutions.

   B. This indicator primarily addresses
      ☐ a process of patient care.
      ☒ a patient outcome.

IV. RATIONALE
   A. Excessive maternal blood loss represents a patient outcome which may suggest the need for further review. This indicator assesses practitioner judgment and technical skill relative to the management of delivery and the immediate postpartum period. It also reflects the comprehensiveness of prenatal and postpartum monitoring.

   B. Selected references:
      American College of Obstetricians and Gynecologists: Diagnosis and management of postpartum hemorrhage. *ACOG Technical Bulletin*, Washington, DC 1990.   *(continued)*

Obstetrical Care Indicator Development Form (continued)

Cunningham FG, MacDonald PC, Gant NF: Chapter 36 in *Williams Obstetrics*. Norwalk, CT: Appleton and Lange, 1989.

Sachs BP, et al: Hemorrhage, infection, toxemia, and cardiac disease, 1954-85: Causes for their declining role in maternal mortality. *Am J Public Health* 78: 671-675.

C. Identify the practitioner and/or organizational processes assessed by this indicator.
   1. Practitioner skill and experience in delivery technique.
   2. Comprehensiveness of prenatal monitoring.
   3. Comprehensiveness of postnatal monitoring.

V. DESCRIPTION OF INDICATOR POPULATION
   A. Subcategories—None

   B. Data Format
      1. Numerator: the number of deliveries with excessive maternal blood loss.
      2. Denominator: the total number of mothers delivered.

VI. REQUIRED DATA ELEMENTS AND LOGIC
   A. Data Elements
      See Addendum "Master Data Element List"

   B. Indicator Logic

OB-3. MATERNAL BLOOD LOSS

IF   **Maternal Diagnosis** =
       placenta previa without hemorrhage (641.0-)
       hemorrhage from placenta previa (641.1-)
       premature separation of placenta, abruptio (641.2-)
THEN   Delete (exclude)
THEN   OB-3 Population = Yes

IF   **Maternal Procedure** =
       autotransfusion of whole blood (99.02)
       other transfusion of whole blood (99.03)
       transfusion of packed cells (99.04)
THEN   OB-3 = YES

IF   **Red Blood Cell Transfusion** = Yes
THEN   OB-3 = Yes

IF   **Postdelivery Hematocrit** < 22
THEN   OB-3 = Yes

IF   **Postdelivery Hemoglobin** < 7
THEN   OB-3 = Yes

IF   **Predelivery Hgb** − **Postdelivery Hgb** ≥ 3.5
THEN   OB-3 = Yes

IF   **Predelivery Hct** − **Postdelivery Hct** ≥ 11.0
THEN   OB-3 = Yes

(continued)

Obstetrical Care Indicator Development Form (continued)

REPORT:

% of all mothers with excessive maternal blood loss = $\dfrac{\text{Sum of OB-3}}{\text{Total mothers delivered}}$

VII. UNDERLYING FACTORS
   A. Patient-based factors (ie, factors outside the healthcare organization's control contributing to patient outcomes)
      1. Maternal
         a. Coagulation disorder
         b. Preexisting anemia
      2. Fetal/Infant
      3. Other patient factors (ie, nondisease factors which may have an impact on care—eg, age, sex, refusal of consent)
         a. Compliance with prenatal care instructions

   B. Non–patient-based factors (ie, factors within the healthcare organization's control or problem areas causing indicator activity)
      1. Practitioner technical skill in delivery technique
      2. Practitioner knowledge and judgment related to intrapartum monitoring and management
      3. Continuity of care
      4. Communication and coordination with ancillary services

FIGURE 4.B. *Figure 4.A. filled out for one of the Joint Commission's recommended obstetrics indicators, "Maternal blood loss."*

Indicator Worksheet

Department/Unit _____

Important Aspect of Care/Service:

_____

_____

_____

_____

Indicator Category:

_____

_____

_____

Indicator _____

_____

_____

Outcome [ ]   Process [ ]

Perspective: [ ] Customer   [ ] Supplier

Criteria: (if applicable to a process)

_____

_____

_____

Threshold for Evaluation	_____ %	Applied to Aggregate?	____Yes ____No
	Sentinel [ ]	Applied to Individuals or Events?	____Yes ____No
	Comparative [ ]		

Source or Rationale for Criteria/Threshold: _____

_____

_____

Data Collection:

a. Data Source: _____

b. Method: _____

c. Frequency: _____

d. Sample: [ ] Yes   [ ] No

   If yes, state sample size: _____

   and method: _____

Data Comparison Frequency: _____

Data Reporting:

a. Frequency: _____

b. Where: _____

Figure 4.C. *Indicator development worksheet.*
Source: *Evangelical Health Systems, Oak Brook, IL. Used with permission.*

Indicator Proposal Worksheet

Part A. Instructions

Date: (Date report is prepared)
Committee: (Unit where monitor is to be
               conducted)
Department: Clinical Nursing Department

I.   Topic
     • brief explanation of indicator to be
       evaluated
     • how indicator was chosen
     • who identified indicator (ie, individual,
       professional, committee).

II. Objectives of indicator
     • define rationale of indicator
     • measurable, specific.

III. Parameters of monitor
     • person conducting monitor
     • population/sample and how selected
     • size of sample
     • age range (if applicable)
     • sex (if applicable)

     • service (if applicable)
     • unit (if applicable)
     • time period
     • data source
     • data collector
     • frequency of data collection
     • cost
     • describe how data were collected
     • attach a copy of data collection tool.

IV. Action plan
     • action: develop objectives to deal with
       changes in practice that should result
     • responsible individuals: designate person or
       persons and/or committees to review
       findings and incorporate change in practice.

V.   Signatures
     • To occur in order listed. Facilitates
       communications about proposal and
       findings.

Part B. QA Indicator Proposal Format

Date: Theoretical Framework:
Committee:
Department:
Topic:

Objective of Monitoring: Method of Assessment:

                                    _____
                                    Initiator   Date

Methods of Data Collection: _____
                                    Head Nurse (if applicable)   Date

                                    _____
                                    Departmental QA Chairperson   Date

                                    _____
                                    Departmental Clinical Director Date

                                    _____
                                    Coordinator of Quality Assurance Date

Figure 4.D. Indicator proposal form.

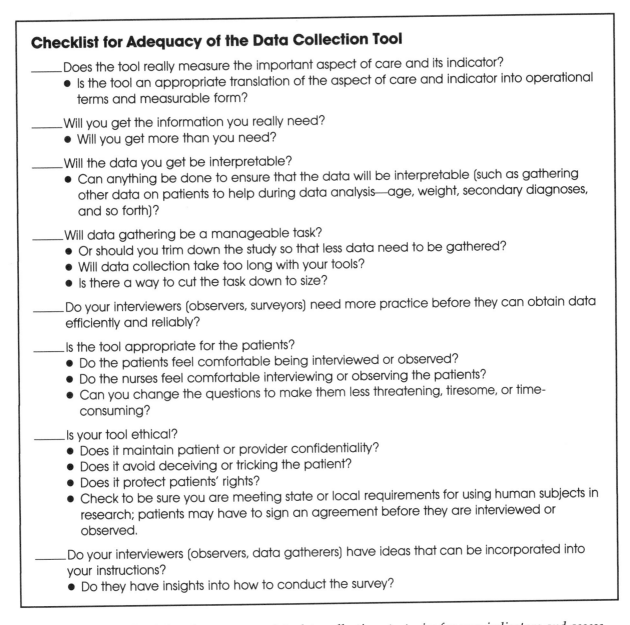

Checklist for Adequacy of the Data Collection Tool

_____Does the tool really measure the important aspect of care and its indicator?
   ● Is the tool an appropriate translation of the aspect of care and indicator into operational terms and measurable form?

_____Will you get the information you really need?
   ● Will you get more than you need?

_____Will the data you get be interpretable?
   ● Can anything be done to ensure that the data will be interpretable (such as gathering other data on patients to help during data analysis—age, weight, secondary diagnoses, and so forth)?

_____Will data gathering be a manageable task?
   ● Or should you trim down the study so that less data need to be gathered?
   ● Will data collection take too long with your tools?
   ● Is there a way to cut the task down to size?

_____Do your interviewers (observers, surveyors) need more practice before they can obtain data efficiently and reliably?

_____Is the tool appropriate for the patients?
   ● Do the patients feel comfortable being interviewed or observed?
   ● Do the nurses feel comfortable interviewing or observing the patients?
   ● Can you change the questions to make them less threatening, tiresome, or time-consuming?

_____Is your tool ethical?
   ● Does it maintain patient or provider confidentiality?
   ● Does it avoid deceiving or tricking the patient?
   ● Does it protect patients' rights?
   ● Check to be sure you are meeting state or local requirements for using human subjects in research; patients may have to sign an agreement before they are interviewed or observed.

_____Do your interviewers (observers, data gatherers) have ideas that can be incorporated into your instructions?
   ● Do they have insights into how to conduct the survey?

FIGURE 4.E. *Checklist helps choose appropriate data collection strategies for new indicators and assess the adequacy of patient satisfaction surveying. This checklist can also be used when actually collecting data (Step 6) to reevaluate data sources and data-collection method.*
SOURCE: *Nursing Quality Assurance Management Learning System, American Nurses' Association:* Guide for Nursing Quality Assurance Coordinators and Administrators. *American Nurses' Association and Sutherland Learning Associates, Inc, 1982.*

Practitioner Clinical Assessment Form

INDICATOR STATEMENT: **1(PH):** Trauma patients with prehospital emergency medical services scene times greater than 20 minutes.

1. Please circle any terms in the indicator statement that are in need of further definition or are unclear.

2. Based on the intent of this indicator, to what degree does this indicator address an aspect of patient care worth monitoring?

Low		Medium		High	No Opinion
1	2	3	4	5	9

3. To what extent do you believe this indicator would flag cases caused primarily by patient factors?

Rarely		Sometimes		Always	No Opinion
1	2	3	4	5	9

4. How often would findings from this indicator raise good questions for use in monitoring and evaluation activities?

Rarely		Sometimes		Always	No Opinion
1	2	3	4	5	9

5. Do you already monitor this indicator or have a similar monitoring activity for this aspect of patient care?

[ ] Yes (Answer A)   [ ] Don't Know (Answer B)   [ ] No (Answer B)

   A. If you responded Yes, has it been useful to monitor?

Not Useful				Very Useful	No Opinion
1	2	3	4	5	9

   B. If you responded Don't Know or No, would it be useful to monitor?

Not Useful				Very Useful	No Opinion
1	2	3	4	5	9

6. To what extent does the rationale adequately express the intent of the indicator?

Poorly				Clearly	No Opinion
1	2	3	4	5	6

7. Additional comments about this indicator:

_____
PROFESSIONAL SPECIALTY

FIGURE 4.F. *The Joint Commission's form for initial rating of the clinical relevance of proposed indicators. This form is sent to surveyed physicians along with a detailed description of the proposed indicator (ie, its rationale, components of care assessed by the indicator, definition of terms, and references from the literature supporting the indicator).*

Medication Use Task Force Rating of Potential Medication Use Indicators (Second Round) Rating Form

Instructions: *Before scoring* please refer to the previous page for definitions of each criteria and review the indicator development form for the indicator being assessed. Please read the indicator statement and rate it with a score of (1) low to (5) high according to each criteria arrayed at the right. Please make any comments you would like to make on the margin under the indicator. If you feel you need more information to rate an indicator adequately, then please check the *no rating* space below the indicator statement.

NOTE: If an indicator has more than one numerator or denominator, please indicate which one you rated.

Scoring
5 = high
4 = high/medium
3 = medium
2 = medium/low
1 = low

INDICATOR STATEMENT	CRITERIA					COLLECTIBILITY				
	Importance to Patient Outcome	Problematic Area	Utility for Improving Patient Care	Definitional Clarity	Availability of Data	Numerator Size	Difficulty/Complexity of Data Collection	Benefits vs Effort of Data Collection	Variability of Data Collection Methods	Risk Adjustment
MU-1 Indicator (Numerator): Inpatients receiving one or more doses of H$_2$ blockers _____ No rating										
MU-2 Indicator (Numerator): Inpatients >65 years old in whom creatinine clearance has been estimated _____ No rating										
MU-2a Indicator (Numerator): Patients under 1 year old receiving aminoglycosides in whom creatinine clearance has been measured _____ No rating										

FIGURE 4.G. The Joint Commission's ''second-round'' indicator rating form (used after Figure 4.F.), sent to practitioners shortly before field testing the indicators. The overall purpose of second-round rating of potential indicators is to determine: (1) indicators that are ready for testing (with minor revisions), (2) indicators that need further Task Force discussion and major revisions before testing, and (3) indicators that the Joint Commission should not pursue further. This second round of rating focuses on the collectibility of data.

Worksheet for Testing Indicators

Answer each question for each of your drafted indicators.

Is It VALID?

1. Does the indicator need to be further validated because it represents a new concept or procedure in nursing care, because it's controversial, or because it includes specific numerical values that may be questionable?
   Further validation needed for indicator #:
   __, __, __, __, __, __

2. Does the indicator really respond to the priority issues in the important aspects of care? Does it measure what it's intended to measure? Is it low priority? Does it suggest that other indicators are missing?
   Eliminate low priority indicator #:

   __, __, __, __, __, __

   Gaps still exist; write indicator for the following issues:

   _____

   _____

3. Does the indicator fit the important aspect of care? Does it apply to all patients and providers included in the population in question? Is it appropriate for the data-gathering methods selected (eg, questionnaire, observation, record review)?
   Eliminate indicator #: __, __, __
   Modify indicator #: __, __, __

4. Does the indicator represent an important issue to nurses or will it seem trivial? Is it consistent with important nursing values?
   Eliminate indicator #: __, __, __
   Modify indicator #: __, __, __

Is It MEASURABLE?

5. Is the indicator stated in measurable terms? Are behavioral terms, operational definitions, numerical values, specific terms, and clarifying notes included wherever possible?

   Eliminate indicator #: __, __, __
   Modify indicator #: __, __, __

6. Are there predictable exceptions to this indicator other than those you've already incorporated in writing it? Can you think of other patient conditions, nursing diagnoses, provider behaviors, situations, or interventions that are appropriate exceptions? (Don't bother to include obvious exceptions unless a non-nurse will be gathering the data.)
   Write additional exceptions for indicator #: __, __, __, __, __, __
   Exceptions: _____

   _____

   _____

7. Does the indicator measure just one thing? Is it singly focused? If not, can it be split into several single-issue indicators?
   Write single-focused indicators to replace indicator #: __, __, __, __

Is It APPROPRIATE?

8. Will the indicator be acceptable to those nurses whose practice is being evaluated? Do they need to be (further) involved in development of the indicator? Are they likely to question the appropriateness of the indicator? Do you think they will have revisions to suggest?
   Ratify indicator #: __, __, __, __, __, __

9. Is it feasible? Do you have the resources to collect and analyze the data? Does the study involve a great deal of nurses' time? Are patients' rights or comfort involved in the monitor?
   Eliminate indicator #: __, __, __
   Modify indicator #: __, __, __

FIGURE 4.H. A worksheet designed to support the testing of indicators for validity, measurability, and appropriateness. The form allows space for noting indicators that fail to meet each criterion.
SOURCE: Adapted from Nursing Quality Assurance Management Learning System. American Nurses' Association: Workbook for Nursing Quality Assurance Committee Members: General Practice in Acute Care Hospitals. American Nurses' Association and Sutherland Learning Associates, Inc, 1985.

Clinical Indicators of Quality

RATING SCALE: 5 . . . 1 (5 = very often or more than 75% of the time to 1 = very seldom or unlikely)

Clinical Indicator	Does the provider play a *MAJOR* role in the outcome (as measured by the indicator)	Can a threshold for evaluation be defined?	Is comparative data available?	Is the data financially feasible to collect?	Does the severity of the patients' illness have no effect on results?

FIGURE 4.I. *Worksheet for rating the usefulness of proposed clinical indicators.*
SOURCE: *Spath PL: Consider many factors when developing clinical quality indicators.* Hospital Peer Review *13(9):109, Sept 1988.*

Sample Test Site Questionnaire for Assessment of Indicator Utility

Purpose of Questionnaire: To obtain feedback on the experience of indicator testing to date. Responses are essential for assessing indicators' utility for presentation to the task force and the board of the organization developing the indicators.

GENERAL QUESTIONS TO TEST SITES:

1. Data gathered through the indicators have been shared or utilized by the following (check those that apply):

   Quality Assurance   _____
   Risk Management   _____
   Hospital Administration   _____
   Hospital Medical Staff   _____
   Departmental Committee   _____
   Not shared to date   _____
   Other (please describe)   _____

   Comments:

2. Prior to participating as a test site, was the health care organization monitoring indicators similar to or exactly the same as any of the current indicators? If yes, please describe which indicators and by whom.

3. Has participating in this project resulted in any changes in the health care organization, for example, instituted new data collection systems, improved patient care documentation, changed data on patterns of practice, improved quality assurance activities? If yes, please describe.

4. Describe positive and/or negative aspects of participating in this project.

INDICATOR-SPECIFIC QUESTIONS:

A. Overall ease of data collection for this indicator:
   Very Easy   Very difficult   Not applicable
       1   2   3   4   5   N/A

B. How useful is this indicator in monitoring processes/outcomes?
   Not useful   Very Useful   Not applicable
       1   2   3   4   5   N/A

FIGURE 4.J. *Questionnaire used by test site staff members to assess the utility of the Joint Commission's indicators.*

Sample Test Site Individual Case Assessment Form

Medical Record Number _____

Reviewer Title (eg, MD, RN) _____

Indicator (eg, maternal excessive blood loss): _____

1. Should this medical record have been flagged for further review? Was it reasonable for you to review this record, regardless of your ultimate conclusions about it?

   _____ NO _____ YES   If NO, please explain _____
   _____
   _____

2. Based on your review of this case, do clearly documented patient factors (eg, severity of illness, comorbidity, or other factors *not* within the practitioner or hospital's control) explain why this indicator flagged this case?

   _____ NO
   _____ YES, completely explained
   _____ YES, partially explained

   If YES, what is this patient factor(s)? _____
   _____
   _____

3. Listed below are the components of care this indicator is likely to monitor. Based on your review of this medical record, which components are related to why this case was flagged by this indicator? Please circle all that apply or add in "other" component not mentioned.

   A. Practitioner judgment and capability related to the management of the patient care activity assessed by the indicator (eg, second and third phases of labor)
   B. Clinical staff's capability related to the above
   C. Organization systems' problems; please describe:
   _____
   _____
   D. Other: _____
   E. Documentation in medical record limits assessment

4. What areas of care might be identified as presenting opportunities for improvement and what improvements would you recommend? _____
   _____

5. Additional comments: _____
   _____

FIGURE 4.K. The Joint Commission's form used by hospital staff members at indicator test sites to assess individual cases flagged by indicators undergoing field testing. Case review may lead to identification of additional important quality-of-care issues and improvement opportunities not directly related to the event targeted for monitoring by the indicator.

Three-Part Indicator Rating System

PART 1. INDIVIDUAL TOPIC PRIORITY WEIGHTS

Institution: _____ Team Member Initials: _____ Date: _____

Instructions:

1. Using a scale of 1 through 5 (5 = high), weight the potential improvement for proposed indicators for clinical relevance and data collectibility within acceptable resource constraints (such as cost and time).

2. After group discussion for *each* topic, immediately record any revision of your item weight in the right column.

Collation Topic	Initial Weights	Revised Weights	Collation Topic	Initial Weights	Revised Weights
A	_____	_____	K	_____	_____
B	_____	_____	L	_____	_____
C	_____	_____	M	_____	_____
D	_____	_____	N	_____	_____
E	_____	_____	O	_____	_____
F	_____	_____	P	_____	_____
G	_____	_____	Q	_____	_____
H	_____	_____	R	_____	_____
I	_____	_____	S	_____	_____
J	_____	_____	T	_____	_____

(continued)

Three-Part Indicator Rating System (continued)

PART 2. COLLATION FORM FOR PRIORITY TOPIC WEIGHTS

Topic	Weight* 5	4	3	2	1	Final Score† (Total of All Weights)
A						
B						
C						
D						
E						
F						
G						
H						
I						
J						
K						
L						
M						
N						
O						
P						
Q						
R						
S						

*Tabulate weights using a single mark to represent an individual vote for a single weight. For example,

Topic A =　$\dfrac{5}{I}$　$\dfrac{4}{JHt}$　$\dfrac{3}{}$　$\dfrac{2}{II}$　$\dfrac{1}{I}$

indicates one 5, five 4's, no 3's, two 2's and one 1.

†Compute final score by multiplying each weight by total marks for that weight and then adding all totals. For example, from above, $(5 \times 1) + (4 \times 5) + (2 \times 2) + (1 \times 1) = 30$.

(continued)

Three-Part Indicator Rating System (continued)

PART 3. PRIORITY TOPIC SUMMARY LIST

Facility: _____ Date: _____

Topic	Initial Weight	Total	Second Weight	Total
A	WT: 5 4 3 2 1 #: =		WT: 5 4 3 2 1 #: =	
B	WT: 5 4 3 2 1 #: =		WT: 5 4 3 2 1 #: =	
C	WT: 5 4 3 2 1 #: =		WT: 5 4 3 2 1 #: =	
D	WT: 5 4 3 2 1 #: =		WT: 5 4 3 2 1 #: =	
E	WT: 5 4 3 2 1 #: =		WT: 5 4 3 2 1 #: =	
F	WT: 5 4 3 2 1 #: =		WT: 5 4 3 2 1 #: =	

FIGURE 4.L. *Three-part format in which practitioners can record their weighting of proposed indicators before and after group discussion. One way to move toward consensus—and elicit expert opinion—is to use such a modified Delphi survey method. Part 2 is a collation form for priority weights, and Part 3 a summary list of priority weights.*
SOURCE: *Adapted from Williamson JW, Ostrow PC, Braswell HR:* Health Accounting for Quality Assurance. *Rockville, MD: American Occupational Therapy Association, 1981, pp 92-94.*

Acute Tonsillitis, Payne: Hawaii Study

INTERNAL MEDICINE PANEL

I. Services recommended
  A. History: specific reference to: *Weight*
     1. Onset   1.0
     2. Duration   1.0
     3. Chills and/or fever   1.0
     4. Previous episodes   1.0
     5. Rheumatic fever or nephritis   1.0
     6. Pain in throat   1.0
     7. Systemic symptoms   1.0
  B. Physical examination: specific reference to:
     1. Appearance of pharynx   3.0
     2. Cervical lymph nodes   2.0
     3. Ears   0.5
     4. Nose   0.5
     5. Chest   1.0
     6. Heart murmur   2.0
     7. Temperature   2.0
     8. Pulse   1.0
     9. Abdominal examination for splenomegaly   1.0
    10. General appearance   1.0
  C. Laboratory
     1. Throat culture for streptococcus   3.0
  D. Therapy
     1. If streptococcus tonsillitis, penicillin (or erythromycin)   3.0

PEDIATRICS PANEL

I. Services recommended
  A. History: specific reference to:
     1. Onset and duration of illness   2.0
     2. Contact history (similar illness in family or associates)   3.0
     3. Duration and degree of fever (patient feels hot!)   1.0
     4. Symptoms of coryza   2.0
     5. Symptoms of laryngitis   2.0
     6. Symptoms of anorexia   1.0
     7. Symptoms of rash (dermatitis)   3.0
     8. Gastrointestinal symptoms   2.0
     9. Previous treatment and response   3.0
     The panel predicted that the record will show only "sore throat and fever of 2-3 days
     duration," but that the foregoing history will have been obtained.
  B. Physical examination (until age 14 years) specific reference to:
     1. General appearance   3.0
     2. Temperature   2.0
     3. Weight   1.0
     4. Examination of oral cavity   3.0
     5. Lymph nodes in general, with emphasis on cervical nodes   2.0
     6. Eyes, ears, nose   3.0
     7. Chest by auscultation   0.5
     8. Heart: auscultation, apical impulse   0.5

(continued)

Acute Tonsillitis, Payne: Hawaii Study (continued)

	Weight
9. Abdomen: palpation of liver and spleen	2.0
10. Fontanelle, if present	1.0
11. Neck suppleness	1.0
12. Skin	3.0
13. Extremities	0.5

The panel predicted that, even when a thorough examination is made, the record will show only the appearance of the tonsils and tympanic membranes, temperature (for patients over 5 years old, observations of a heart murmur or of spleen size may be included).

C. Laboratory

Throat culture for streptococcus screening	3.0

FIGURE 4.M. *Elements of care for acute tonsillitis weighted by a group of physicians for importance ("3" indicating the greatest importance noted); this sort of weighting can be done in preparation for identifying the most important elements of care to monitor.*
SOURCE: *Payne BC, et al:* The Quality of Medical Care: Evaluation and Improvement. *Chicago: Hospital Research and Educational Trust, 1976, pp 133-134. (adapted in Donabedian A:* Explorations in Quality Assessment and Monitoring, Volume II: The Criteria and Standards of Quality. *Ann Arbor, MI: Health Administration Press, 1982, pp 419-421).*

Clinical Indications for Carotid Endarterectomy: A Comparison of Panelists' Ratings and Published Recommendations (1977 through 1981)

Endarterectomy should be performed if the patient has the presentation	ARTICLES[a]			PANEL	
	NUMBER				
	Yes	No	Rank[b]	Rating[c]	Order
Carotid Transient Ischemic Attack(s)	14	0	1	7.5	1
Completed Mild Stroke	6	0	2	7.2	2
Asymptomatic	15	4[d]	3	5.0	3
Asymptomatic, Other Surgery Planned	14	4[d]	4	4.1	4
Stroke-in-evolution	3	4	5	4.3	5
Vertebrobasilar TIAs	0	8[d]	6	3.1	6

a) 88 articles were reviewed; 46 had recommendations for or against carotid endarterectomy.
b) Based on percent of articles endorsing each general clinical presentation.
c) Average median of panel's ratings across 16 identical indications: 1 = very inappropriate; 5 = equivocal; 9 = very appropriate.
d) Either no, or "medical therapy should be tried first."

FIGURE 4.N. *Results of panelists' ratings of the importance of clinical indications for carotid endarterectomy. The table includes a comparison of panelists' ratings and published recommendations. The ranking of indicators by the panelists was nearly identical to that found in the literature.*
SOURCE: *Merrick NJ, et al: Derivation of clinical indications for carotid endarterectomy by an expert panel.* Am J Public Health *77(2):189, Feb 1987.*

Drug Usage Evaluation Topic Planner

Important Aspect of Care (List overall clinical, pharmacy, or laboratory procedures that warrant formal evaluation because they may be inadequate or staff compliance may need improvement)	Evaluating Now?		High Priority?			
	Yes	No	No	Yes		
				Initiate	Continue As Is	Revise
Accuracy of prescription filling and dispensing	X				X	
Availability of emergency drug supplies		X	X			
Appropriate preparatory instructions given to patients undergoing creatinine clearance studies		X	X			
Handling of telephone calls from patients who have problems with prescribed medications	X					X
Completeness of prescriptions		X		X		
Maintenance of accurate patient prescription files	X				X	

Figure 4.O. This form helps staff determine which important aspects of care are being monitored through use of indicators, and facilitates prioritization of aspects of care for future monitoring. **Source:** *Adapted from Joseph ED, Brown R, Celestin C:* Protocols for Evaluating Ambulatory Care, Volume 2: Drug Usage Evaluation. *Chicago: Care Communications, 1988, p 34.*

Quality Assurance Indicator Evaluation

Department ___Radiology___   Aspect of Care ___Accuracy of Diagnosis___

Date _____

A	B	C*	D†	E
List current indicators.	Has current indicator been effective? Yes/No	Has current indicator identified problems? Yes/No	If problems have been identified, have they been resolved? Yes/No	List those indicators to be implemented or continued in next quarter.
Disagreements between radiologist's diagnosis and pathology reports, endoscopy findings, autopsies, or pulmonary function studies.				
Missed diagnoses for lung and breast cancer.				
Missed diagnoses for bone fractures.				
Disagreements between initial interpretation and second independent interpretation by professional peer.				
Percentage of positive biopsies for breast lesions detected by mammography.				

*If no problems have been identified, indicator may be inappropriate.
†If column D is answered "No," continue to use indicator but reevaluate action taken to resolve problem.

FIGURE 4.P. *Form helps staff evaluate indicators in use.*
SOURCE: *Adapted from Gray CS: Quality assurance in a rehabilitation facility: A decentralized approach. QRB 14:9-14, Jan 1988.*

Obstetrical Care Indicator Abstract

I. INDICATOR

OB-3. MATERNAL BLOOD LOSS

Patients with excessive maternal blood loss defined by intra and/or postpartum red blood cell transfusion or a low postdelivery hematocrit or hemoglobin (Hct < 22%, Hgb < 7 gms) or a significant pre- to postdelivery decrease in hematocrit ($\geq$ 11%) or hemoglobin ($\geq$ 3.5 gms) excluding patients with abruptio placenta or placenta previa.

II. DEFINITION OF TERMS

Predelivery Hgb/Hct: the most recent Hgb or Hct value within one week prior to delivery.

Postdelivery Hgb/Hct: the lowest value recorded subsequent to delivery and prior to hospital discharge.

Transfusion includes:
autotransfusion of whole blood (99.02)
other transfusion of whole blood (99.03)
transfusion of packed cells (99.04)

Primary Exclusion Criteria:
If maternal diagnosis:
placenta previa without hemorrhage (641.01)
hemorrhage from placenta previa (641.11)
premature separation of placenta, abruptio (641.21)

III. RATIONALE

Excessive maternal blood loss represents a patient outcome which may suggest the need for further review. This indicator assesses practitioner judgment and technical skill relative to the management of delivery and the immediate post-partum period. It also reflects the comprehensiveness of prenatal and post-partum monitoring.

IV. USE OF INDICATOR BY HOSPITAL

This is a rate-based indicator: further assessment by the hospital is warranted if the occurrence rate shows a noticeable trend over time or indicates statistically significant differences when compared to peer institutions.

Numerator: the number of deliveries with excessive maternal blood loss.

Denominator: the total number of mothers delivered.

V. SELECTED REFERENCES

American College of Obstetricians and Gynecologists: Diagnosis and management of postpartum hemorrhage. *ACOG Technical Bulletin,* Washington, DC 1990.

Cunningham FG, MacDonald PC, Gant NF: Chapter 36 in *Williams Obstetrics.* Norwalk, CT: Appleton and Lange, 1989.

Sachs BP, et al: Hemorrhage, infection, toxemia, and cardiac disease, 1954-85: Causes for their declining role in maternal mortality. *Am J Public Health* 1988, 78: 671-675.

FIGURE 4.Q. The Joint Commission's format for recording indicator parameters and data elements (in this case for the indicator "Maternal Blood Loss," used as an example in Figure 4.B.).

Form for the Description of Indicators

Department/service:

Important aspect of care:

Indicator:

Exceptions to indicator:

Type of indicator (process or outcome):

Threshold for evaluation:

Data source:

Definitions and instructions for data retrieval (eg, what specific information, number, or other identification is needed?):

Person responsible for data collection/tabulation:

Data collection frequency:

Sample size:

Instructions for sampling:

Exclusions from sample:

Frequency of data tabulation and comparison to threshold for evaluation:

Person responsible for evaluation when threshold reached:

Content and frequency of summary reports:

Criteria proposed to evaluate summary data and initiate further investigation:

Figure 4.R. Form for the description of indicators.

Examples of Clinical Indicators

HOSPITALWIDE	CROSS-DEPARTMENTAL	SPECIALTY-SPECIFIC
For general application:	**For surgical departments:**	**For obstetrics departments:**
• Nosocomial infection rates	• Complications of surgery	• Delivery of infant < 1800 grams in hospitals without an NICU
• Deaths	• Discrepancies between preop diagnosis and pathology findings	• Hyaline membrane disease after elective C-section
• Pressure ulcers		
• Complications resulting from medication errors	**For medical departments:**	• In-hospital initiation of antibiotics 24 hours or more following term vaginal delivery
	• Drug interactions and reactions	• Apgar $\leq$ 3 at 5 minutes
	• Complications of IV and other lines	• Neonatal mortality in infants 750-1000 grams in hospitals with an NICU

FIGURE 4.S. Matrix to group indicators by whether they apply to hospitalwide, cross-departmental, or specialty-specific issues.

Identifying Problem Areas in Your Facility

DEPARTMENT/SERVICE _____

Considering the information presented in this chapter, think about problems that might exist in your facility and complete the following exercise on problem identification.
1. Note five problems that you suspect exist in your facility.
2. For each suspected problem, list all data sources that might help verify its existence.
3. For each suspected problem, note the ways in which patient care might be affected adversely.
4. Note potential explanations for the existence of each problem.

SUSPECTED PROBLEMS	PROBLEM INDICATORS	DATA SOURCES	IMPACT ON PATIENT CARE	POTENTIAL EXPLANATIONS	SUGGESTED SOLUTIONS

How does the suspected problem affect patient care or outcome?

How many patients would be affected adversely by the suspected problem?

What clinically valid indicator would be used to measure compliance with expected performance?

Is the problem resolvable?

How difficult or costly would it be to conduct a formal assessment of the problem?

FIGURE 4.T. *Opportunities to improve or problems may be apparent in aspects of care and service that are not being monitored with indicators. (Leaders and others in the organization must establish channels—eg, surveys, complaints, suggestions—by which they receive feedback that is not part of ongoing monitoring, but that is related to the quality of care and service.) In these cases, the monitoring and evaluation process may be bypassed and the situation evaluated to determine how to improve and to guide actions to be taken. This form is designed for listing such opportunities to improve and establishing the order in which they will be addressed.*

Identifying Data Sources in Your Facility

For each of the data sources listed, identify whether it is available in your facility, whether it is currently used to identify problems, and which quality assurance (QA) functions in your facility use or could use information generated by the data source.

Data Source	Available Yes No	Currently Used Yes No	QA Function
Patient record review			
Morbidity/mortality review			
Patient care monitoring (individual case review)			
Monitoring activities of clinical and other professional staffs			
Findings of committee activities			
Review of prescriptions			
Incident reports relating to safety and to clinical care			
Review of laboratory, radiologic, and other diagnostic clinical reports of services rendered			
Financial data			
Utilization review findings			
Data from staff interviews and observations of patient services			
Patient surveys or comments			
Management information system data			
Consumer complaints			
Annual reports			
Response to crises			
Trustee complaints			
Profile analyses			
Third-party payers/fiscal intermediaries reports			
Literature review			
Research studies			
JCAHO survey recommendations			
Computerized data reports			
Tissue review			
Blood utilization review			
Safety committee findings			
Infection control committee findings			
Liability claims data			

FIGURE 4.U. *Many existing data sources can be used in monitoring and evaluation. This form helps remind those developing indicators of some of the data sources that can be tapped.*

Excerpts from Abstraction Guidelines for Diabetes Mellitus*

Item	Indicator Description	Definition	Location in the Chart	Acceptable or Equivalent Statements
1	FPG ≥ 150 mg/dl	Fasting plasma glucose	A lab finding; may be recorded on chemistry report or in the body of the encounter	Record positive if: FPG ≥ 150 mg/dl Record negative if: FPG done, but values not ≥ 150 mg/dl Record absent if: There is no mention of FPG
9	Taking insulin/ oral agents	Patient currently takes insulin or another hypoglycemic agent (drug used to lower blood sugar)	Subjective findings (history)—with statements about current medications, or in some treatment plan prior to date	Record positive if: patient takes: Insulins: regular, Semilente®, lente, globin, NPH®, PZI, Ultralente® Oral agents: Orinase® (tolbutamide), Diabinese® (chlorpropamide), Dymelor® (acetohexamide), DBI® (phenformin), Tolinase® (tolazamide) Record negative if: patient takes: no medications; patient takes a list of medications not including above

*FPG = fasting plasma glucose

FIGURE 4.V. Excerpt from guidelines on abstracting data from the medical record concerning diabetes mellitus. "Record positive" refers to words or values in patient records that conform in meaning with the indicator. The final column provides interpretations of alternative statements that may be found in the medical record. Stipulating statements in patient records that are equivalent to the indicator may be part of formulating the indicator.
SOURCE: Graham NO: Quality Assurance in Hospitals: Strategies for Assessment and Implementation. Rockville, MD: Aspen Systems Corp, 1982, p 153.

Data Collection/Review/Display

DIRECTIONS: Considering the indicators you have already developed, identify the following:

1. Individual Responsible for Data Collection
   Indicator #1 _____
   Indicator #2 _____
   Indicator #3 _____
   Indicator #4 _____

2. Frequency of Collection
   Indicator #1 _____
   Indicator #2 _____
   Indicator #3 _____
   Indicator #4 _____

3. Sample Size
   Indicator #1 _____
   Indicator #2 _____
   Indicator #3 _____
   Indicator #4 _____

4. What data source will be utilized
   Indicator #1 _____
   Indicator #2 _____
   Indicator #3 _____
   Indicator #4 _____

FIGURE 4.W. Simple form for showing the data collection plan for each indicator monitored.
SOURCE: Ravenswood Hospital Medical Center, Chicago. Used with permission.

Patient Satisfaction Questionnaire

1. Prior to this hospitalization, about how many times have you been admitted to a hospital and stayed one or more nights?
   [ ] never
   [ ] one other time
   [ ] two other times
   [ ] three or more other times

2. Have you ever been hospitalized at Brigham and Women's Hospital before?
   [ ] yes   [ ] no

3. For most of your stay, were you in your room alone or with other patient(s)?
   [ ] alone in a room
   [ ] in a room with other patient(s)

4. Before you came to the hospital, did your doctor tell you how long you would be here?
   [ ] yes   [ ] no

5. How long did you think you would be in the hospital?
   minimum days: _____   maximum days: _____

6. What additional information would you have liked prior to your hospitalization?
   Comments: _____

ADMISSION

7. When you were admitted, did anyone offer to answer any questions you had about payment?
   [ ] yes   [ ] no

8. When you were admitted, how long was it between the time you arrived and the time you were actually in your room?
   minutes: _____   hours: _____

9. If there were any delays, did the admitting staff explain the reason for those delays?
   [ ] yes   [ ] no   [ ] no delays

PLEASE RATE THE FOLLOWING ASPECTS OF YOUR CARE
(Circle one answer)

	Excellent	Very good	Good	Fair	Poor
ADMITTING STAFF					
10. Explanation of financial issues by admitting staff	5	4	3	2	1
11. Courtesy and helpfulness of admitting staff	5	4	3	2	1
Comments: _____					
NURSES					
12. Courtesy and helpfulness of your nurses	5	4	3	2	1
13. The nurses' efforts to answer questions and keep you informed	5	4	3	2	1
14. How quickly the nurses took care of your needs	5	4	3	2	1
15. Overall, the skill of the nurses who cared for you	5	4	3	2	1
Comments: _____					

(continued)

Patient Satisfaction Questionnaire (continued)

DOCTORS	Excellent	Very good	Good	Fair	Poor
16. Courtesy and helpfulness of your doctors	5	4	3	2	1
17. The doctors' efforts to answer questions and keep you informed	5	4	3	2	1
18. Doctors' explanations of tests or operations	5	4	3	2	1
19. Overall, the skill of the doctors who cared for you	5	4	3	2	1

Comments: _____

YOUR ROOM					
20. Cleanliness and comfort of your room	5	4	3	2	1
21. Working condition of appliances in your room (eg, bed, sink, blinds)	5	4	3	2	1
22. Television service	5	4	3	2	1
23. The ease of finding your way around the hospital	5	4	3	2	1

24. What suggestions do you have for improving the rooms in the hospital?

Comments: _____

RADIOLOGY (X-RAY) TESTS DURING YOUR HOSPITALIZATION

25. Did you have an x-ray or CT scan while you were in the hospital?
    [ ] yes   [ ] no   [ ] don't know
    If yes, how long did you have to wait at the x-ray department before being seen?
    Minutes: _____

FOOD AND NUTRITION SERVICES	Excellent	Very good	Good	Fair	Poor
26. Courtesy of food service staff	5	4	3	2	1
27. Quality of food, compared to other hospitals or cafeterias	5	4	3	2	1

Comments: _____

DISCHARGE

28. How efficiently was your discharge handled?   5   4   3   2   1
29. Did a nurse explain what to expect and how to care for yourself after discharge?
    [ ] yes   [ ] no
30. Did a doctor explain what to expect and how to care for yourself after discharge?
    [ ] yes   [ ] no
31. Were your concerns about posthospital care addressed early in your stay?
    [ ] yes   [ ] no
32. Overall, is your health better or worse than you expected it to be at this point?

Much better	Somewhat better	What I expected	Somewhat worse	Much worse
5	4	3	2	1

33. Do you feel that you are "back to normal"?
    [ ] yes   [ ] no
    If no, how many days do you think it will be until you feel normal again?
    Number of days: _____

Comments: _____

(continued)

Patient Satisfaction Questionnaire (continued)

34. Would any of the following services have been helpful to you in your recovery at home? (Check all that apply.)

[ ] Equipment   [ ] Housekeeping services
[ ] Follow-up phone call from hospital nurse   [ ] Registered nurse home visit
[ ] Other (please specify):
_____

35. How would you describe the length of your hospital stay?

[ ] A lot shorter than I needed   [ ] A little longer than I needed
[ ] A little shorter than I needed   [ ] A lot longer than I needed
[ ] About right

36. Why did you come to Brigham and Women's Hospital for your hospitalization? (Please check the most important reason.)

[ ] Hospital reputation   [ ] Telephone yellow pages
[ ] Friend's recommendation   [ ] Transferred from another hospital
[ ] My physician is on staff   [ ] Television, newspaper, or radio
[ ] Outside physician referral   advertisement
[ ] Other (please describe below): [ ] Ambulance brought me
_____

37. Would you recommend the hospital to your friends and family?

[ ] yes   [ ] no

Overall rating of hospital	Excellent	Very good	Good	Fair	Poor
38. Overall satisfaction with stay	5	4	3	2	1

Comments: _____

Optional background information

39. Which of the following income categories best describes your total 1987 household income?

[ ] $7,500 or less   [ ] $25,001 to $50,000
[ ] $7,501 to $25,000   [ ] $50,001 or more

40. Which of the following terms best describes your ethnic background?

[ ] Black   [ ] Oriental
[ ] White   [ ] Other
[ ] Hispanic

41. Please add any additional comments about your hospitalization that you wish to make. We would especially like to know what you liked most and least about your stay.

Figure 4.X. Patient satisfaction survey administered to selected medical patients in a hospital. *Source:* Brigham and Women's Hospital, Boston. Used with permission.

Child/Parent Questionnaire

FOR KIDS ONLY

You were a patient at Children's Hospital not long ago. We would like to know how you felt about being in the hospital. The answers you give to these questions will help us make the time spent in the hospital more comfortable and pleasant for all children. Color in the face that tells us your feelings. Ask your mother or father for help with the questions, if you need it.

On the way to the hospital, I felt:	happy	afraid	sad	angry
While I was in the hospital, I felt:	happy	afraid	sad	angry
On the way home, I felt:	happy	afraid	sad	angry

The nurses were:	great	ok	ugh
The doctors were:	great	ok	ugh

DEAR PARENTS:

We are pleased that your child is able to return home now and the entire staff of Children's Hospital of Wisconsin joins in wishing you well.

We would be very appreciative if you would return the attached questionnaire at your earliest convenience. We have included a patient's page for those children old enough to respond.

ABOUT YOUR CHILD

Age _____ Nursing Unit/Floor _____ Zip Code (home) _____
Date of Admission _____ Date of Discharge _____
Did your child have a pre-admission tour? _____Yes _____No

ABOUT ADMISSION

1. Were admitting personnel helpful and courteous?
   _____Yes _____No _____Somewhat

2. Were you given a parent handbook?
   _____Yes _____No

(continued)

Child/Parent Questionnaire (continued)

ABOUT ADMISSION (continued)

3. If there was a delay in admission, was the reason explained to you?
   _____Yes _____No
   Additional Comments: _____
   _____
   _____

ABOUT PATIENT CARE

1. Did a nurse see your child promptly after admission to the patient room?
   _____Yes _____No

2. Did you feel the nursing care met your child's needs?
   _____Yes _____No _____Somewhat

3. Was the nursing staff understanding of your needs as parents of a sick child?
   _____Yes _____No _____Somewhat

4. Did you know who your child's physician was?
   _____Yes _____No _____Not Sure

5. Did your child's physician give an adequate explanation of your child's condition?
   _____Yes _____No _____Somewhat

6. Did you have to ask or remind the doctor or nurses of necessary care for your child?
   _____Sometimes _____Seldom _____Never
   Additional Comments: _____
   _____
   _____

ABOUT FOOD

1. Within the restrictions of diet ordered by your physician, did your child enjoy his food?
   _____Always _____Usually _____Seldom

2. Was your child's menu accurately served?
   _____Always _____Usually _____Seldom

ABOUT THE HOSPITAL

1. Your general impression of the hospital was:
   _____Excellent _____Good _____Fair _____Poor

2. Was your child's room neat and clean?
   _____Yes _____No

3. Did you have any difficulty finding the visitor parking lot?
   _____Yes _____No

4. Did you have any difficulty finding CHW?
   _____Yes _____No _____Somewhat

(continued)

Child/Parent Questionnaire (continued)

ABOUT THE HOSPITAL (continued)

5. If it were necessary for your child to return to a hospital, would you choose Children's Hospital?
_____Yes _____No
Additional Comments: _____
_____
_____

ABOUT OUR SERVICES

Many other people may have helped care for or performed services for you or your child. If you would like to let us know about your experience, please comment:
_____
_____
_____

ABOUT DISCHARGE & BILLING

1. Your discharge process was handled:
_____Promptly _____Routinely _____Slowly

2. If you had trouble understanding items on your bill, were the items explained in a helpful manner?
_____Yes _____No _____Does Not Apply

3. Additional Comments: _____
_____

What was the most difficult thing for you during the time your child was in the hospital?
_____
_____
_____

Date: _____

Child's Name _____
OPTIONAL

Parent's Name _____
OPTIONAL

Address _____
OPTIONAL

FIGURE 4.Y. *Satisfaction survey for children (and their parents) cared for in a hospital.*
SOURCE: *Children's Hospital of Wisconsin, Milwaukee. Used with permission.*

Patient Satisfaction Survey Questionnaire for an Ambulatory Care Center

The "Give Us A Grade" patient satisfaction questions:

THE FACILITY

Card 1. Give us a grade for:

Clean building:	A B C D F
Easy to find where to go:	A B C D F
Rooms neat, picked up:	A B C D F
Comfort while here:	A B C D F

THE APPOINTMENT PROCESS

Card 2. Give us a grade for:

Getting an appointment to see the doctor:	A B C D F
How nice the appointment people were:	A B C D F

WAITING TIME

Card 3. Give us a grade on your wait after you got here:

In the waiting room:	A B C D F
In the exam room:	A B C D F

THE FISCAL PROCESS

Card 4. Give us a grade on:

What you pay to see the doctor:	A B C D F
How clear the bill was:	A B C D F
The way we collect money:	A B C D F

SATISFACTION WITH STAFF

Card 5. Give our doctor a grade on:

Understanding what you said:	A B C D F
Taking enough time with you:	A B C D F
Telling you what you needed to know:	A B C D F
Being careful and helpful:	A B C D F

Card 6. Give our nurse a grade on:

Understanding what you said:	A B C D F
Taking enough time with you:	A B C D F
Telling you what you needed to know:	A B C D F
Being careful and helpful:	A B C D F

Card 7. Give our medical assistant a grade on:

Understanding what you said:	A B C D F
Taking enough time with you:	A B C D F
Telling you what you needed to know:	A B C D F
Being careful and helpful:	A B C D F

Card 8. Give our receptionist a grade on:

Understanding what you said:	A B C D F
Taking enough time with you:	A B C D F
Telling you what you needed to know:	A B C D F
Being careful and helpful:	A B C D F

Card 9. Give our cashier a grade on:

Understanding what you said:	A B C D F

(continued)

Patient Satisfaction Survey Questionnaire for an Ambulatory Care Center (continued)

Taking enough time with you: A B C D F
Telling you what you needed to know: A B C D F
Being careful and helpful: A B C D F

Satisfaction with Health Outcome

Card 10. Give us a grade for how much better your health is
          after you come to the health center: A B C D F

Participation in Development of Health Care Plan

Card 11. Give our doctor and staff grades for:

Listening to you: A B C D F
Using your ideas: A B C D F
Taking your way of living into plans for your health: A B C D F

Patient Education Activity

Card 12. Give us a grade for teaching you about new medicines:

How to use them: A B C D F
What to expect from them: A B C D F
Give us a grade for teaching you about NEW things to
   do at home to help your health (things like soaking
   foot, exercise and special diet):   A B C D F

Card 13. Give us a grade for:

Teaching you about how to take care of your health: A B C D F
How helpful the handouts are in understanding your health
   care plan: A B C D F

Card 14. Give us a grade for how well our doctor or nurse taught you:

About your condition: A B C D F
What your medicine is for: A B C D F
How to take your medicine: A B C D F
What to do for better health: A B C D F

Patient Concerns Understood by Physician

Card 15. Give us a grade for how well the doctor understood you: A B C D F

Patient Compliance

Card 16. Give **YOURSELF** a grade for:

Doing what the doctor and nurse told you to do the last
   time you were here: A B C D F
Taking your medicine as directed: A B C D F
Coming back when the doctor told you: A B C D F

Card 17. Has the doctor told you to change any of your health
          habits (like: smoking, drinking, exercise, diet, cancer
          check, safety or other)?   Yes No

If yes, give yourself a grade for how well you are doing: A B C D F

Trust in Health Care Staff

Card 18. Give us a grade for how easy it is to tell the doctor things
          that are hard to talk about: A B C D F

Card 19. Give us a grade to show how much you feel the staff
          cares about you and your health: A B C D F

(continued)

Patient Satisfaction Survey Questionnaire for an Ambulatory Care Center (continued)

Card 20: Give us a grade to show how much you feel you can trust the staff (not counting the doctor):   A B C D F

Card 21. Give us a grade on how much you feel you can trust your doctor: A B C D F

NEW PATIENTS

Card 22. Were you given a New Patient Handbook today?   Yes No

If you were very sick when you called to make an appointment, were you able to see the doctor within 24 hours?   Yes No

If you needed an appointment for regular health care, were you able to see the doctor within 7 days after you called?   Yes No

ACCESSIBILITY

Card 23. If you are very sick, were you able to see the doctor within 24 hours after you called?   Yes No

If you came in for regular health care, were you able to see the doctor within 48 hours of the time you wanted?   Yes No

Card 24. Give us a grade for:

When you need to reach the doctor or nurse, how easy is it for you to talk with them on the day you call?   A B C D F

Card 25. Give us a grade for:

How easy it is to reach a health center doctor any time of the day or night when someone is sick or hurt: A B C D F
OR CHECK ONE:
_____ never tried   _____ did not know I could

Card 26. How did you get to the health center (Circle all that apply):

bus	friend's car
walk	cab
your car	other

Give us a grade for how easy it is for you to get to the health center: A B C D F

Card 27. How did you first hear about the health center (Circle all that apply):

family	TV
friend	Silver Pages
newspaper	Outreach
poster	NeighborHealth
radio	Other

AVAILABILITY

Card 28. Give us a grade on how well you like the clinic hours: A B C D F

(continued)

Patient Satisfaction Survey Questionnaire for an Ambulatory Care Center (continued)

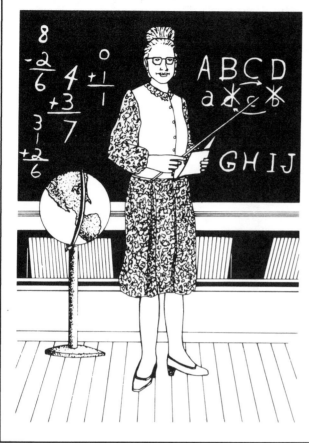

GIVE US A GRADE

12. Give us a grade for teaching you about new medicines:

How to
use them: A   B   C   D   F

What to expect
from them: A   B   C   D   F

Give us a grade for
teaching you about
NEW things to do at
home to help your health
(things like soaking
foot, exercise and
special diet):   A   B   C   D   F

FIGURE 4.Z. *Patient satisfaction survey developed by an ambulatory care center. The "Give Us a Grade" Satisfaction Forms are a series of 25 cards (see example above) distributed to patients after treatment. The form as printed here is a compilation of the questions printed on those cards.*
SOURCE: *Community Health Network, Inc, and Methodist Hospital of Indiana, Inc, Community Health Centers, Indianapolis. Used with permission.*

Thank You

for choosing Saint Elizabeth Community Health Center for your health care services. To help us better serve you in the future, please take a few minutes to complete and return this short survey.

Overall, how would you rate the quality of care you received at Saint Elizabeth?

Excellent	Good	Fair	Poor
4	3	2	1

Will you choose Saint Elizabeth for future health care needs?

☐ Not likely   ☐ Somewhat likely   ☐ Very likely

If you checked "Not likely," please let us know why you would not choose Saint Elizabeth and/or how we can improve our services

_____

_____

_____

_____

_____

Date of Visit _____

Comments

_____

_____

_____

_____

_____

I would like to be contacted by hospital management to discuss my care.

☐ Yes   ☐ No

Name _____ Phone _____

(optional)

Figure 4.AA. Brief hospital patient satisfaction questionnaire.
Source: Marker J: Integrating patient satisfaction into your QA/RM program—or, pleased patients seldom sue. Journal of Quality Assurance 10(5):10, Dec/Jan 1989.

Telephone Interview Script

SCRIPT	RESPONSE
Hello, patient's name. My name is Henry Wodsworth and I am the administrator of the radiology department at General Hospital.	SMILE!
If it is convenient for you, and you feel well enough, I was wondering if you would be willing to spend 5 or so minutes with me on the telephone so that I might be able to learn of your impressions and opinion of the services we delivered to you on an outpatient basis on day?	Pause for response If not convenient, ask if you can call back. If not interested, thank the caller.
Thank you very much. Do I understand correctly: Dr _____ is the physician who ordered your scan?	_____ Yes _____ No
M _____, did you personally make the appointment, or did Dr _____'s receptionist make it for you?	_____ Patient _____ Doctor _____ Don't remember
Did the receptionist who scheduled the procedure explain where our department was located in the hospital? (and offer to give you directions to the hospital)?	_____ Yes _____ No _____ Don't remember
Did she verify our billing policy over the phone and request that you bring all of your insurance information?	_____ Yes _____ No _____ Don't remember
Did you encounter any problems finding our department once you were in the hospital?	_____ Yes _____ No
When you arrived, did our receptionist greet you in a warm and friendly manner?	_____ Yes _____ No _____ Don't remember
Did our receptionist introduce herself to you? Do you remember her name?	_____ Yes _____ No _____ Don't remember _____ Receptionist's name
Do you remember whether she called you by name?	_____ Yes _____ No _____ Don't remember
Did the receptionist explain that the radiologist would send a separate bill to you?	_____ Yes _____ No _____ Don't remember
Can you estimate how long you had to wait between the time you registered and the time one of our technicians came out and escorted you back into the dressing room where you changed your clothes?	_____ Less than 5 minutes _____ 5-10 minutes _____ 11-20 minutes _____ 21-30 minutes _____ Over 30 minutes _____ Don't remember *(continued)*

Telephone Interview Script (continued)

SCRIPT	RESPONSE
Did you feel that amount of time was excessive?	_____ Yes _____ No _____ No opinion
I do know that on _____, about the time you were scheduled, we had several other unexpected procedures come up, which created delays. Did the receptionist alert you to the delay and estimate how long the wait might be?	_____ Yes _____ No _____ Don't remember
Did the technician introduce herself to you?	_____ Yes _____ No _____ Don't remember
Did she call you by name?	_____ Yes _____ No _____ Don't remember
Did she explain, to your satisfaction, the procedure before she began?	_____ Yes _____ No _____ Don't remember
Do you remember whether she asked you if you had any questions?	_____ Yes _____ No _____ Don't remember
If you had any questions, did you feel the technician did a good job of answering those questions?	_____ Yes _____ No _____ No opinion
Do you feel the technician was gentle in handling you during the procedure?	_____ Yes _____ No _____ No opinion
Once you were done, did the technician tell you what to anticipate as far as expelling the barium we injected?	_____ Yes _____ No _____ Don't remember
I have just two more questions, M _____. Overall, did you feel that the staff was responsive to your needs?	_____ Yes _____ No _____ No opinion
Is there anything we could have done to make the procedure easier for you?	
Thank you for your time, M _____. Do you have any other questions I can answer?	

FIGURE 4.BB. *Interview script for a patient satisfaction survey conducted by telephone.*
SOURCE: *Peterson K:* The Strategic Approach to Quality Service in Health Care. *Rockville, MD: Aspen Publishers, 1988, pp 175-176.*

Department of Radiology Patient Questionnaire

Please complete this survey form. If it is not picked up from you personally, when it is completed, either return it to the front x-ray desk, or mail it to us.

Your comments will help us in our continual effort to provide the best possible x-ray service. Thank you!

WAITING TIME:

Even the simplest of x-ray examinations may require you to be in the X-Ray Department for at least half an hour. Obviously, the more complex examinations require a longer time. Based on what you were told, do you feel your stay in the X-Ray Department exceeded the necessary time period?

Yes ☐   No ☐   Comments: _____

How long would you say you were in the X-Ray Department?

30 Minutes _____   One Hour _____

Two Hours _____   Longer (please specify)
_____
_____

TYPE OF EXAMINATION:

_____
_____
_____
_____
_____
_____

COURTESY AND THOUGHTFULNESS:

Check the following which best describes the manner in which you were treated while in the X-Ray Department:

_____ Unsatisfactory   _____ Below Average

_____ Average   _____ Very Good

Outstanding _____

Was the nature of your x-ray examination explained to you previously by:

Your physician   ☐ Yes   ☐ No
The technologist   ☐ Yes   ☐ No

Effort on the part of the x-ray personnel to inform you of the nature of your x-ray examination and what would be expected of you during the procedure:

_____ Unsatisfactory   _____ Below Average

_____ Average   _____ Very Good

_____ Outstanding

ADDITIONAL COMMENTS:

In the space below, we would appreciate hearing from you in regard to any comments you might have about our X-Ray Department:

_____
_____
_____

FIGURE 4.CC. *Survey instrument to measure patient satisfaction with services provided by a hospital radiology department.*
SOURCE: Q.A. Guide: Appropriateness in Patient Care Services. *Reston, VA: American College of Radiology, 1983, p 22.*

Patient Meal Survey

This survey is being conducted four times a year as part of a continuing effort to provide you with satisfactory food service. Your cooperation in completing this questionnaire will be most appreciated.

To complete, please answer the following questions by marking an X in the section that best describes your opinion of that aspect of the food service.

	Excellent	Very Good	Good	Fair	Poor
1. How acceptable is the appearance and aroma of the food?					
2. How clean are the dishes and the silverware? (If meal service uses disposable ware, please go on to question #3)					
3. How is the temperature of the hot foods?					
4. How do you rate the variety of the food?					
5. How satisfactory are the portion sizes of your food?					
6. How do you rate the flavor of the foods served to you?					
7. How is the temperature of the cold foods?					
8. When you receive your meals, are they complete and accurate as expected?					
9. What is your overall rating of this Food Service?					

10. Has a representative of the Dietetics Department discussed your food service or nutritional care?

Yes _____   No _____

11. Do you fill out your menu daily?

Yes _____   No _____

12. How long have you been in the hospital?

Less than 4 days _____   More than 4 days _____

13. What kind of diet are you on? _____

14. Do you have an adequate understanding of the diet you will need to follow at home?

We welcome your comments and suggestions for improvements in food service: _____

_____

_____

_____

Figure 4.DD. Form to measure patient satisfaction with hospital food service.
Source: Marriott Quality Improvement Manual, *Washington, DC: Marriott Corp, 1990, p 71.*

Checklist for Patient's Perception of Nursing Care

HOSPITAL NAME AND ADDRESS

TO OUR PATIENTS:

Today this hospital is making a study to find out how to give *better nursing care* to you, and to all patients in the future.

On the following pages we have listed things that may have happened to you while you have been here. We are asking all patients who are well enough to *help the hospital* and *help the nurses* by checking these items.

1. Read each item carefully.

2. If something *did happen* today, put a check in the box that says, "This happened today." If it did *not* happen today, but *did* happen some other day *during this stay* in the hospital, put a check in the box that says, "This happened some other day." (You may have to check both boxes in some cases.)

If it *did not happen* during this stay in the hospital, then check the box that says, "This did *not* happen."

3. Do not sign your name.

4. Put your completed form in the envelope and seal it.

5. If there is something you want to say that is not included, please write it on the last page.

Please be frank. Your frank answers added to all other patients' will help the hospital get more help for our nurses.

PATIENTS: PLACE CHECK MARKS IN APPROPRIATE BOXES FOR ALL STATEMENTS	DURING MY PRESENT STAY IN THIS HOSPITAL		
	THIS HAPPENED TODAY	THIS HAPPENED SOME OTHER DAY	THIS DID NOT HAPPEN
1 Radio or TV noisy	✔	✔	
(Examples) If a radio or TV was noisy today, you would check "this happened today." If noisy some other day *during your present stay* in this hospital, you would check "this happened some other day." If noisy *both* today and some other day, you would check *both* boxes.			
2 My bath was not given on time.			✔
If your bath was always given on time during your *present stay* in this hospital, you would check this statement in the third box.			
3 Couldn't get anything from the nurse for pain.			
4 My call for a nurse was answered very promptly.			
5 Food trays left in front of me too long.			
6 Thermometer left in too long.			
7 No answer to call for a nurse for a long time.			

(continued)

Checklist for Patient's Perception of Nursing Care (continued)

PATIENTS: PLACE CHECK MARKS IN APPROPRIATE BOXES FOR ALL STATEMENTS	DURING MY PRESENT STAY IN THIS HOSPITAL		
	THIS HAPPENED TODAY	THIS HAPPENED SOME OTHER DAY	THIS DID NOT HAPPEN
8 Bedpan was handled too noisily.			
9 Bedpan was left with me too long.			
10 Nurse or aide didn't leave me clean towels.			
11 Food was served in a hurry.			
12 Drinking water wasn't changed.			
13 Other patients made disturbing noises.			
14 Nurse left before I could ask her questions.			
15 Had to wait too long for a bedpan.			
16 My nurse left me alone too long when I was allowed up.			
17 There was no one to feed me when I needed help.			
18 Room was too chilly or too warm to sleep.			
19 Not propped up, making it hard to enjoy my meal.			
20 My nurse explained my care to me.			
21 Nurse wanted me to do too much for myself.			
22 I was not bathed as thoroughly as I would like.			
23 Light was too bright when I tried to sleep.			
24 There was too much noise in the hall.			
25 Nurses didn't seem interested in me.			
26 Bathroom was not clean.			
27 Radios, TV's or record players were played too loudly.			
28 Bed was not made right.			
29 My bath, meal or rest period interrupted by treatment.			
30 Had to get out of bed to take a bath even though I felt bad.			
31 Woken up too early for temperature taking.			
32 Was not served milk or fruit juice after I requested it.			
33 Room in general was not made neat and orderly.			
34 My nurse is always in a hurry.			
35 My nurse wouldn't tell me what was wrong with me.			
36 My food was cold when served.			

(continued)

Checklist for Patient's Perception of Nursing Care (continued)

PATIENTS: Place Check Marks In Appropriate Boxes For All Statements	During My Present Stay In This Hospital		
	This Happened Today	This Happened Some Other Day	This Did Not Happen
37 My nurse did not tell me anything about my treatment.			
38 My nurse was especially nice to me.			
39 Had to wait a long time to use the bathroom.			
40 Nurse was unfriendly.			
41 Didn't see a nurse often enough.			
42 Bed was not changed when needed.			
43 Nurse did not wash and rub my back well.			
44 Air in room was poor.			
45 Didn't get my medicine until late.			
46 My aide is always in a hurry.			

Some of the following statements could have happened only to some people. Please check any statement that applies to you. Leave the others blank:

47 My bandage or dressing was too tight.			
48 No one checked needle in my arm to see that fluid was running.			
49 I was not told when I would be operated on.			
50 Asked for a wheelchair and didn't get one.			
51 Asked for a heat lamp but I never got it.			
52 My bed got wet from treatment.			

Additional Comments:

Figure 4.EE. *Checklist for a patient's perception of nursing care. This checklist asks patients to remember occurrences of annoying or less than adequate care.*
Source: Instruments for Measuring Nursing Practice and Other Health Care Variables, Volume 2, Health Manpower Reference Series, DHEW Pub. No. 78-54.

Concurrent Patient Interview Questionnaire

Interviewer: _____

Date Due: _____

Patient Room: _____ Length of Stay: _____

Objectives: a) To evaluate the extent to which patients are satisfied with selected aspects of nursing care.

b) To evaluate the extent to which patients identify/experience specific characteristics of Primary Nursing.

Directions:

- Review the Interview Questions prior to beginning your interview (to familiarize yourself with the questions and new format).
- Interview 1 patient on _____ .
- Interview a patient who has been hospitalized for a *minimum of 48 hours.* Interview a patient who is alert and oriented—or if patient is unable to respond appropriately, family members who are closely involved with patient and staff may be interviewed.
- Utilize the patient's Medical Record, Nursing Care Plan and Primary Nurse Board to complete Length of Stay and Part II, DOCUMENTATION.
- Complete your interview by the date due indicated above and return to your Unit Supervisor.
- If the patient identifies significant concerns when interviewed, discuss them immediately with the Primary Nurse, Quad Clinician, Unit Supervisor or Unit Director.

I. PATIENT INTERVIEW

A. Questions:	Yes	No	Comments
1. Do you have a nurse taking care of you who introduced herself/himself to you as your Primary Nurse?			
2. Do you have a nurse who cares for you on a consistent basis?			
3. Has your Primary Nurse/one of the nurses discussed your care plan (including your concerns about your hospitalization) with you?			
4. Has she/he discussed your discharge with you? Any changes in your usual daily activities after this hospitalization?			
5. Do you feel you have the information you need (to care for yourself/be cared for) to go home?			

(continued)

Concurrent Patient Interview Questionnaire (continued)

B. Questions:	75-100% Yes-Usually	50-74% Occasionally	25-49% Sometimes	0-24% Rarely-No	Comments:
1. Does the nurse taking care of you (for day and PM shifts) introduce herself/himself to you at the beginning of the shift?					
2. Do you feel that the nurses taking care of you are genuinely concerned about you? (as a person; about your condition, comfort)					
3. Have the nurses been available when you've needed something? (the bathroom, pain relief, water/food, change of position)					
4. Do you feel confident in the nurses taking care of you? Their skill, knowledge, ability?					
5. Do you feel that the nurses respect you as a person?					
6. Do you feel the nurse is available to spend time with you (as needed)? (to listen, to talk, to help with problems/concerns)					
7. Have the nurses helped you get the rest/sleep you need to get well?					
8. Do the nurses explain things (the usual routines and any tests or procedures you've had) in terms you can understand?					

II. Documentation	Yes	No	Comments
1. Primary Nurse is indicated on Primary Nurse Board.			
2. Primary Nurse is indicated on Nursing Care Plan (care plan, not patient care routines).			
3. The Primary Nurse has cared for the patient _____ days since admission (review graphic record for signatures).			

Figure 4.FF. *Form to record patient responses during a face-to-face interview concerning quality of nursing care.*
Source: *St Mary's Hospital, Milwaukee. Used with permission.*

Patient Problem Report

Date _____

Patient's name _____

Patient's record number _____ Room no. _____ Phone no. _____

Patient's home address and home phone number

_____

(Address)

_____

(City, state, zip code)

_____

(Phone)

Describe patient's problem or concern. Be specific. Note when, how, from whom you learned of
the problem. _____

_____

_____

_____

List other persons, services, or departments involved. _____

_____

_____

Describe action taken to solve problem. _____

_____

_____

_____

FIGURE 4.GG. *Form to record the details of a patient problem or complaint, and what was done about it.*
SOURCE: Patient Representation in Contemporary Health Care. *Chicago: American Hospital Association, 1985.*

Patient Representative Monthly Activity Report

Month of _____ , 19___

INQUIRY DATA

Source of inquiry. Record total number of inquiries received from each group listed.

Patient _____
Employee _____
Family or friend _____
Physician _____
Other _____

Mode of inquiry. Record total number of inquiries received via each of the following.

Telephone _____
Letter _____
Interview _____
Page or beeper _____
Other _____

PATIENT PROBLEM AREA DATA

Record the total number of patient problems occurring in each of the following areas.

	Inquiries this month		Inquiries this month
Accounts receivable	_____	Lost and damaged property	_____
Administration	_____	Nursing	_____
Admitting	_____	Occupational therapy	_____
Billing or charges	_____	Parking	_____
Business office	_____	Physical therapy	_____
Community relations	_____	Physician	_____
Coronary care unit	_____	Pulmonary laboratory	_____
Diet—food	_____	Recovery room	_____
Diet—instructions	_____	Respiratory therapy	_____
Diet—tray delivery	_____	Roommate or room problem	_____
Discharge	_____	Social services	_____
Electrocardiogram (EKG)	_____	Speech therapy	_____
Electroencephalogram (EEG)	_____	Surgery	_____
Emergency department	_____	Translation	_____
Employee attitude	_____	Transportation	_____
Engineering	_____	Ultrasound	_____
Environmental services	_____	X-ray	_____
Financial counseling	_____	Other (specify)	_____
Gastrointestinal laboratory	_____	_____	
Hemodialysis	_____	_____	
Intensive care unit	_____	_____	
		Total	_____

_____
Guest Relations Rep. Signature

FIGURE 4.HH. *A monthly summary report of patient problems or complaints, with the number of problems tabulated by category. The same type of material could be presented in an annual summary, with vertical columns showing number of problems per month in each category.*
SOURCE: *Sinai Hospital, Detroit. Used with permission.*

Mystery Visitor Evaluation

Date: _____ "Mystery Visitor" _____

UNIVERSITY HOSPITAL & CLINIC
STANDARDS OF HOSPITALITY AND CARING

Philosophy of Caring

We believe in the dignity and worth of all individuals, including those who serve as well as those who are served, and strive to achieve excellence in care through the principles of courtesy, respect, and concern. We are proud of our institution, our professions, and our service to others.

Area Visited:

1. What was the approximate time of your visit?
2. Was the area busy at the time of your visit?
3. How long did you have to wait before someone offered assistance?
4. How many people did you approach for help?
5. Were you able to identify people by UNHC name badges or some other form of ID?
6. Were the individuals you approached:

   - Professionals (ie, nurses, doctors, etc)
   - Clerical (ie, receptionists, secretaries, etc)
   - Service (ie, maintenance, food service, etc)?

7. Were you treated with courtesy and respect?
8. Did anyone interrupt their work or go out of their way to help you?
9. If directions were given, were they clear and understandable?
10. Rank the areas you visited on a scale of 1–3 with 1 being given to the area where you felt someone best demonstrated the Philosophy of Caring.

In your opinion, who is the one individual you encountered during your visit who best demonstrated the Philosophy of Caring to you?

Are there any comments you would like to make regarding your experience with this project?

FIGURE 4.II. *Structure to guide the impressions of a "mystery visitor" hired to visit the hospital and rate its service.*
SOURCE: *University Hospital, University of Nebraska Medical Center, Omaha. Used with permission.*

Questionnaire for Physicians Outside the Radiology Department Regarding X-Ray Services

1. What is the quality of the x-ray film? excellent _____ good _____ satisfactory _____ needs improvement _____ . If satisfactory or needs improvement, what are some of the problems with the films? _____
   _____
   _____

2. How would you rate the present quality of x-ray reports? excellent _____ good _____ satisfactory _____ needs improvement _____ . If satisfactory or needs improvement, what are some of the problems? _____
   _____
   _____

3. How would you rate the turnaround time of reports? excellent _____ good _____ satisfactory _____ needs improvement _____ . If satisfactory or needs improvement, what are some of the problems? _____
   _____
   _____

4. Have you ever experienced a delay in fluoroscopy or intravenous pyelogram (IVP) scheduling? Yes _____ No _____ . If yes, how often would you say this delay happens? _____
   _____
   _____

5. What could be done to improve x-ray service to you?
   _____
   _____
   _____

6. Other comments:
   _____
   _____
   _____

FIGURE 4.JJ. Questions for physicians outside the radiology department regarding their satisfaction with radiology services.
SOURCE: Batalden PB, O'Connor JP: Quality Assurance in Ambulatory Care. Germantown, MD: Aspen Systems Corp, 1980, p C:11.

Nurses' Questionnaire on Patients' Bill of Rights

	Do you agree with this statement?			Is this statement true in this hospital?		
	Yes	No	Undecided	Yes	No	Undecided
1. The patient has the right to considerate and respectful care.						
2a. The patient has the right to obtain from his physician complete current information concerning his diagnosis, treatment, and prognosis in terms the patient can be reasonably expected to understand.						
2b. When it is not medically advisable to give such information to the patient, the information should be made available to an appropriate person in his behalf.						
2c. He has the right to know by name the physician responsible for coordinating his care.						
3a. The patient has the right to receive from his physician information necessary to give informed consent prior to the start of any procedure and/or treatment.						
3b. Except in emergencies, such information for informed consent should include but not necessarily be limited to the specific procedure and/ or treatment, the medically significant risks involved, and the probable duration of incapacitation.						
3c. Where medically significant alternatives for care or treatment exist, or when the patient requests information concerning medical alternatives, the patient has the right to such information.						
3d. The patient also has the right to know the name of the person responsible for the procedures and/or treatment.						
4. The patient has the right to refuse treatment to the extent permitted by law, and to be informed of the medical consequences of his action.						

(continued)

Nurses' Questionnaire on Patients' Bill of Rights (continued)

	Do you agree with this statement?			Is this statement true in this hospital?		
	Yes	No	Undecided	Yes	No	Undecided
5a. The patient has the right to every consideration of his privacy concerning his own medical care program. Case discussion, consultation, examination, and treatment are confidential and should be conducted discreetly.						
5b. Those not directly involved in his care must have the permission of the patient to be present.						
6. The patient has the right to expect that all communications and records pertaining to his care should be treated as confidential.						
7a. The patient has the right to expect that within its capacity a hospital must make reasonable response to the request of a patient for services.						
7b. The hospital must provide evaluation, service, and/or referral as indicated by the urgency of the case.						
7c. When medically permissible a patient may be transferred to another facility only after he has received complete information and explanation concerning the needs for and alternatives to such a transfer.						
7d. The institution to which the patient is to be transferred must first have accepted the patient for transfer.						
8a. The patient has the right to obtain information as to any relationship of his hospital to other health care and educational institutions insofar as his care is concerned.						
8b. The patient has the right to obtain information as to the existence of any professional relationships among individuals, by name, who are treating him.						
9a. The patient has the right to be advised if the hospital proposes to engage in or perform human experimentation affecting his care or treatment.						
9b. The patient has the right to refuse to participate in such research projects.						

(continued)

Nurses' Questionnaire on Patients' Bill of Rights (continued)

	Do you agree with this statement?			Is this statement true in this hospital?		
	Yes	No	Undecided	Yes	No	Undecided
10a. The patient has the right to expect reasonable continuity of care.						
10b. He has the right to know in advance what appointment times and physicians are available and where.						
10c. The patient has the right to expect that the hospital will provide a mechanism whereby he is informed by his physician or a delegate of the physician of the patient's continuing health care requirements following discharge.						
11. The patient has the right to examine and receive an explanation of his bill regardless of source of payment.						
12. The patient has the right to know what hospital rules and regulations apply to his conduct as a patient.						

FIGURE 4.KK. *This self-administered questionnaire consists of 25 statements that are designed to provide information on nurses' attitudes toward patients' rights and whether or not these rights are provided for in a particular health care setting.*
SOURCE: Instruments for Measuring Nursing Practice and Other Health Care Variables, Volume 2, Health Manpower Reference Series, DHEW Pub. No. 78-54.

Staff Perceptions Questionnaire

This self-administered questionnaire is part of an overall effort to refine and develop a method for monitoring the quality of nursing care. The questionnaire, aside from asking you for some background information, is concerned primarily with your ideas about nursing. Please answer each question carefully and honestly. If you cannot answer a question, just leave it blank. All answers will be confidential; you will not be identified in any way.

PART 1

Hospital _____

Age _____

On which specific unit do you work?

_____

Type of school in which you received your (basic) nursing education:

_____ Junior college
_____ Hospital
_____ College or university
_____ School of practical nursing

Present position (circle one):

Practical nurse
Staff nurse (RN)
Head nurse
Supervisor
Clinical specialist
Other (please specify): _____

Please list all degrees (most recent first) or diplomas, schools, and year of graduation.

School	Degree	Year
_____	_____	_____
_____	_____	_____
_____	_____	_____
_____	_____	_____

PART 2

This set of questions refers to your evaluation of the work personnel in many departments in this hospital. Please answer each question by circling the response that best indicates your rating of this hospital.

(continued)

Staff Perceptions Questionnaire (continued)

Part 2 (continued)

How well do the different jobs and work activities around the patient fit together to give good patient care? (Circle one.)
1. Perfectly
2. Very well
3. Fairly well
4. Not so well
5. Not well at all

To what extent do the people from the various departments make an effort to avoid creating problems or interfering with one another's work? (Circle one.)
1. To a very great extent
2. To a great extent
3. To a fair extent
4. To a small extent
5. To a very small extent

To what extent are all related things and activities well timed in the everyday routine of the hospital? (Circle one.)
1. Perfectly timed
2. Very well timed
3. Fairly well timed
4. Not so well timed
5. Rather poorly timed

How well planned are the work assignments of the people from the different departments who work together? (Circle one.)
1. Extremely well planned
2. Very well planned
3. Fairly well planned
4. Not so well planned
5. Not well planned at all

In general, how well established are the routines of the different departments that have to work with one another? (Circle one.)
1. Extremely well established
2. Very well established
3. Fairly well established
4. Not too well established
5. Not well established

From time to time changes in policies, procedures, and equipment are introduced by the management. How often do these changes lead to better ways of doing things? (Circle one.)
1. Changes of this kind never improve things.
2. They seldom improve things.
3. About half of the time they do.
4. Most of the time they do.
5. Changes of this kind are always an improvement.

How well do the various persons who are affected by these changes accept them? (Circle one.)
1. Very few of the persons involved accept the changes.
2. Less than half do.
3. About half of them do.
4. Most of them do.
5. Practically all of the persons involved accept the changes.

In general, how do you *now* feel about changes during the past year that affected the way your job is done? (Circle one.)
1. Made things somewhat worse.
2. Did not improve things at all.
3. Did not improve things very much.
4. Improved things somewhat.
5. Have been a big improvement.
6. There have been no changes in my job in the past year.

During the past year when changes were introduced that affected the way your job is done, how did you feel about them *at first*? (Circle one.)
At first I thought the changes would:
1. Make things somewhat worse.
2. Not improve things at all.
3. Not improve things very much.
4. Improve things somewhat.
5. Be a big improvement.
6. There have been no changes in my job in the past year.

(continued)

Staff Perceptions Questionnaire (continued)

PART 3A

For each of the following activities, please circle the appropriate number indicating how often the activities are included in your present position. [Supervisory form: Please circle the appropriate number indicating how often you expect nurses under your leadership to perform each activity in their present positions.]

Activity	Present position		
	Never	Sometimes	Often
1. Transcribing orders to other records (eg, medication cards or Kardex)	1	2	3
2. Answering the telephone	1	2	3
3. Writing nursing care plans	1	2	3
4. Nursing assessment and planning on admission	1	2	3
5. Planning with physicians for patient care	1	2	3
6. Conducting conferences to plan nursing care	1	2	3
7. Talking with patients and/or families about their concerns or care	1	2	3
8. Operational tasks of the unit such as stamping charts or keeping records in order	1	2	3
9. Giving instructions to patients about their roles in their care	1	2	3
10. Coordinating services of nonnursing departments when their personnel are off duty	1	2	3

PART 3B

For each of the following activities, please circle the appropriate number indicating how often you think the activities in an ideal situation should be included in your role. [Supervisory form: Please circle the appropriate number indicating how often in an ideal situation you would want nurses under your leadership to perform each activity.]

Activity	Ideal situation		
	Never	Sometimes	Often
1. Transcribing orders to other records (eg, medication cards or Kardex)	1	2	3
2. Answering the telephone	1	2	3
3. Writing nursing care plans	1	2	3
4. Nursing assessment and planning on admission	1	2	3
5. Planning with physicians for patient care	1	2	3
6. Conducting conferences to plan nursing care	1	2	3
7. Talking with patients and/or families about their concerns or care	1	2	3
8. Operational tasks of the unit such as stamping charts or keeping records in order	1	2	3
9. Giving instructions to patients about their roles in their care	1	2	3
10. Coordinating services of nonnursing departments when their personnel are off duty	1	2	3

(continued)

Staff Perceptions Questionnaire (continued)

PART 4

The following 40 items are possible descriptions of the behavior of your immediate superior in your present position. Each item describes a specific behavior but does not ask you to judge whether the behavior is desirable or undesirable. The only purpose is to make it possible for you to describe the behavior of the nursing leader. In answering each item, please think about the behavior of your immediate superior. Think about how frequently he/she exhibits each behavior, and draw a circle around the appropriate answer. Be assured that ALL ANSWERS ARE CONFIDENTIAL.

	Always	Often	Occasionally	Seldom	Never
1. Sizes up situations quickly and accurately	A	B	C	D	E
2. Lets group members know what is expected of them	A	B	C	D	E
3. Allows the members complete freedom in their work	A	B	C	D	E
4. Is hesitant about taking initiative in the group	A	B	C	D	E
5. Is alert to everything that happens in the group	A	B	C	D	E
6. Encourages the use of uniform procedures	A	B	C	D	E
7. Permits the members to use their own judgment in solving problems	A	B	C	D	E
8. Fails to take necessary action	A	B	C	D	E
9. Is very sensitive to moods and feelings	A	B	C	D	E
10. Tries out his (her) ideas in the group	A	B	C	D	E
11. Encourages initiative in the group members	A	B	C	D	E
12. Lets other persons take away his (her) leadership in the group	A	B	C	D	E
13. Knows how most members will react to a proposal	A	B	C	D	E
14. Makes his (her) attitudes clear to the group	A	B	C	D	E
15. Lets the members do their work the way they think best	A	B	C	D	E
16. Lets some members take advantage of him (her)	A	B	C	D	E
17. Fails to sense what is expected of him (her)	A	B	C	D	E
18. Decides what shall be done and how it shall be done	A	B	C	D	E
19. Assigns a task, then lets the members handle it	A	B	C	D	E
20. Is the leader of the group in name only	A	B	C	D	E
21. Is aware of conflicts when they occur in the group	A	B	C	D	E
22. Assigns group members to particular tasks	A	B	C	D	E
23. Turns the members loose on a job and lets them go to it	A	B	C	D	E
24. Backs down when he (she) ought to stand firm	A	B	C	D	E

(continued)

Staff Perceptions Questionnaire (continued)

Part 4 (continued)

	Always	Often	Occasionally	Seldom	Never
25. Is perceptive in sizing up individuals	A	B	C	D	E
26. Makes sure that his (her) part in the group is understood by the group members	A	B	C	D	E
27. Is reluctant to allow the members any freedom of action	A	B	C	D	E
28. Lets some members have authority that he (she) should keep	A	B	C	D	E
29. Knows what the members are thinking	A	B	C	D	E
30. Schedules the work to be done	A	B	C	D	E
31. Allows the group a high degree of initiative	A	B	C	D	E
32. Takes full charge when emergencies arise	A	B	C	D	E
33. Is totally insensitive to others	A	B	C	D	E
34. Maintains definite standards of performance	A	B	C	D	E
35. Trusts the members to exercise good judgment	A	B	C	D	E
36. Overcomes attempts made to challenge his (her) leadership	A	B	C	D	E
37. Seems to know when trouble is brewing	A	B	C	D	E
38. Asks that group members follow standard rules and regulations	A	B	C	D	E
39. Permits the group to set its own pace	A	B	C	D	E
40. Is easily recognized as the leader of the group	A	B	C	D	E

Part 5

In this section think about your present work. Please indicate how often each statement below is true in your present work by circling *the appropriate response.*

	Always	Often	Occasionally	Seldom	Never
1. There are an adequate number of nurses on this unit to give the kind of nursing care that should be given.	A	B	C	D	E
2. I have responsibility for too many patients.	A	B	C	D	E
3. I have the right amount of responsibility.	A	B	C	D	E
4. The nursing staff is properly organized to give good nursing care.	A	B	C	D	E

(continued)

Staff Perceptions Questionnaire (continued)

Part 5 (continued)

	Always	Often	Occasionally	Seldom	Never
5. The administration in this hospital wants nurses to assume greater responsibility for managerial or clerical duties than for patient care.	A	B	C	D	E
6. The hospital makes certain requirements of the nurse's time that keep her away from patient care.	A	B	C	D	E
7. I find it best not to question those who are in authority.	A	B	C	D	E
8. My job involves more responsibility for keeping the unit running well than for the direct care of patients.	A	B	C	D	E
9. Nurses do not have the authority to make decisions about a patient's care.	A	B	C	D	E
10. I am able to give the kind of nursing care I think nurses should provide.	A	B	C	D	E
11. Nobody except the patient and his family pays much attention to how well I take care of patients.	A	B	C	D	E
12. I am adequately recognized for the quality of care I give.	A	B	C	D	E
13. I want to continue working as a nurse until I retire.	A	B	C	D	E
14. The most important things that happen to me involve my work.	A	B	C	D	E
15. I have other activities more important than my work.	A	B	C	D	E
16. I avoid taking on extra duties and responsibilities in my work.	A	B	C	D	E
17. I would probably keep working even if I didn't need the money.	A	B	C	D	E
18. I used to care more about my work, but now other things are more important to me.	A	B	C	D	E
19. I'm really a perfectionist about my work.	A	B	C	D	E
20. In my job, I feel pressures for better performance over and above what I think is reasonable.	A	B	C	D	E

(continued)

Staff Perceptions Questionnaire (continued)

PART 6

In this section continue to think about your present work. What is it like most of the time? In the blank beside each word given below, please write:

> _1_ for "Yes" if it describes your work (pay, superior, etc)
> _2_ for "No" if it does not describe it.
>
> _____ Leave blank if you cannot decide.

My Work

_____ Fascinating
_____ Routine
_____ Satisfying
_____ Boring
_____ Good
_____ Creative
_____ Respected
_____ Pleasant
_____ Useful
_____ Tiresome
_____ Healthful
_____ Challenging
_____ Frustrating
_____ Simple
_____ Endless
_____ Gives a sense of accomplishment

My Pay

_____ Income adequate for normal expenses
_____ Satisfactory
_____ Barely live on income
_____ Bad
_____ Income provides luxuries
_____ Insecure
_____ Less than I deserve
_____ Highly paid
_____ Underpaid

Promotions

_____ Good opportunity for advancement
_____ Opportunity somewhat limited
_____ Promotion on ability
_____ Dead-end job
_____ Good chance for promotion
_____ Unfair promotion policy
_____ Infrequent promotions
_____ Regular promotions
_____ Fairly good chance for promotions

My Immediate Superior

_____ Asks my advice
_____ Hard to please
_____ Impolite
_____ Praises good work
_____ Tactful
_____ Influential
_____ Up-to-date
_____ Doesn't supervise enough
_____ Quick-tempered
_____ Tells me where I stand
_____ Annoying
_____ Stubborn
_____ Knows job well
_____ Bad
_____ Intelligent
_____ Leaves me on my own
_____ Lazy
_____ Around when needed

My Co-workers

_____ Stimulating
_____ Boring
_____ Slow
_____ Ambitious
_____ Stupid
_____ Responsible
_____ Fast
_____ Intelligent
_____ Easy to make enemies
_____ Praise good work
_____ Talk too much
_____ Smart
_____ Lazy
_____ Unpleasant
_____ Active
_____ Narrow interests
_____ Loyal
_____ Hard to meet
_____ Busybodies

FIGURE 4.LL. *Perception/satisfaction questionnaire for nurses.*
SOURCE: *Haussmann RKD, Hegyvary ST, Newman JF, Jr:* Monitoring Quality of Nursing Care *(Part II), HEW Publication No. (HRA) 76-7 (Public Health Service Contract NO1 NU-24299, Division of Nursing, Health Resources Administration).*

5 Establish Preliminary Thresholds for Evaluation

This step is designed to help staff identify situations in which a monitored important aspect of care or service must be evaluated. The data collected for each indicator cannot alone lead to conclusions about the quality of care and service. To conclude whether actions can or should be taken to improve care or service requires intensive evaluation of the care and service provided.

It is especially important to know when aspects of care and service being monitored by an indicator may require further evaluation. Since there are not enough resources (eg, people, time, money) to improve *everything all* of the time, resources must be focused first on activities that have the greatest impact on patient outcomes. Those activities in most immediate need of intensive evaluation and improvement certainly include those important aspects of care that are not being performed effectively. To alert staff when a monitored important aspect of care is not being performed as expected and requires further evaluation, mechanisms for triggering such evaluation need to be developed. These mechanisms may include the following:

- Setting statistically derived levels (eg, based on calculation of a standard deviation) for a process or outcome that, when breached, suggest that the activity is not being carried out as expected. (This mechanism of setting tresholds and tracking indicator data against them is discussed at length in Appendix C, page 279.)

- Determining certain patterns of occurrences (eg, more adverse drug reactions on weekends than weekdays) or trends (eg, three consecutive months of increasing complication rates for an invasive procedure) that, when they appear, suggest that the activity is not being carried out as expected.

- Establishing, through review of the relevant literature, the "usual" rate for a process or outcome (eg, a surgical wound infection rate of 3 percent), that, when it is exceeded, suggests that the activity is not being carried out as expected. (Of course, staff may also choose to try to do better than average rates suggested by the literature, and therefore set the threshold for evaluation below occurrence rates that the literature suggests are acceptable). Or

- Identifying an individual occurrence (eg, maternal death) that, when this so-called "sentinel event" occurs, suggests that the activity is not being carried out as expected.

These levels, trends, or patterns are sometimes referred to as "thresholds for evaluation"—the points at which indicator data mandate that more in-depth evaluation must occur. An indicator threshold may be defined as the point at which a stimulus (eg, a single rate or patterns in rates) is strong enough to signal the need for response and the beginning of the process of determining why the threshold has been crossed.

For sentinel event indicators, the threshold is 0%; whenever such an event occurs, it must be evaluated. Organization staff may also choose to more intensively evaluate an important aspect of care even when a threshold is not crossed. For example, even if an activity is being carried out as expected, opportunities for improvement may still exist. (In addition, as discussed under Steps 6 and 7, other feedback from staff, patients, or other sources may trigger intensive evaluation.)

When the threshold for evaluation is other than 0% or 100%, it may be necessary to apply the threshold to the data collected not only for the department or medical staff as a whole, but also for each practitioner separately. In this way, patterns of care for individual practitioners can help identify the need to initiate peer review.

When an indicator is developed, a preliminary threshold for evaluation should be set. However, a threshold is never set permanently. Reevaluating and possible resetting thresholds for evaluation should be a cyclic process, occurring at least once a year. Reevaluate a threshold based on pertinent medical literature and other information sources, and based on your organization's experience collecting data on the indicator in question. A desire for constant improvement is another reason for readjusting the threshold for evaluation.

Organizational experience finding that too many irrelevant cases are falling over the threshold is perhaps the most common reason for adjusting thresholds, particularly if no scientific or external data is available. (As a nonmedical example: if you were to set a device on your car's speedometer to buzz whenever you drove faster than 50 miles per hour, you might find the buzzer to be going off too much, to your annoyance. In which case, you might adjust the threshold upward.)

The setting of thresholds (Step 5) is also addressed in many of the forms included under Step 4 (Identifying Indicators). For example, the "existing data bases" section in Figures 4.A. and 4.B. is intended to direct an organization to objective information (eg, national data bases) that could be consulted when setting a threshold for evaluation.

Figure 5.B. indicates how statistically deriving the standard deviation of variation in indicator data may be used in setting thresholds for evaluation and in comparing collected indicator data with those thresholds (the latter being a function of Step 6). For explanation of how to do this yourself, see Appendix C, page 279. Control charts, of which Figure 5.B. is an example, are also briefly addressed in Figure 7.JJ., where this identical graph is reproduced.

Setting Preliminary Threshold for Evaluation and Periodically Reevaluating the Threshold

Date:

Indicator:

Process(es) of care involved: _____

Department(s) involved in aspect or process of care: _____

_____

Expected indicator/threshold type

    Indicate the approach that would be expected in response to this indicator:

        _____ sentinel event indicator: all occurrences warrant review by the hospital.

        _____ rate-based indicator: further assessment by the hospital is warranted if the occurrence rate shows a noticeable trend over time or indicates statistically significant differences when compared to peer institutions.

Preliminary threshold for evaluation: _____

BASIS FOR PROPOSED THRESHOLD

    Support in medical literature (give reasoning and literature citations):

_____

_____

_____

    Support in the facility's or practitioners' experience:

_____

_____

_____

    Support from industry norms or peer institution averages:

_____

_____

_____

    Other support:

_____

_____

_____

(continued)

Setting Preliminary Threshold for Evaluation and Periodically Reevaluating the Threshold (continued)

EVALUATION OF PRELIMINARY THRESHOLD AFTER THREE MONTHS OR LESS OF MONITORING THE INDICATOR

What are initial indicator levels (include dates)? What percentage of cases exceeds the threshold?

_____

_____

_____

Are cases flagged by the threshold mostly relevant?

_____

_____

_____

Do you suspect that too few cases are being flagged by the threshold? Why?

_____

_____

_____

Should the threshold for evaluation remain as it is? Why or why not?

_____

_____

_____

Should the threshold become more stringent in order to spur the facility on to further improve care and service?

_____

_____

_____

On the lines below list current, readjusted threshold. Document periodic reevaluation of the threshold, including dates of reevaluation.

_____

_____

_____

_____

FIGURE 5.A. *Form to guide the preliminary setting of a threshold for evaluation and periodic reevaluation and possible adjustment of the threshold.*

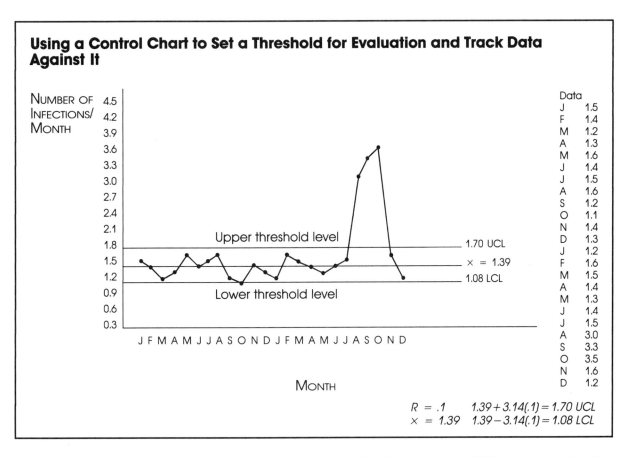

Using a Control Chart to Set a Threshold for Evaluation and Track Data Against It

Figure 5.B. A control chart may be used to set a numerical level for the threshold for evaluation (and to track indicator data to see when the numerical level is crossed). This approach involves calculating the mean and the standard deviation of the mean for a data distribution and then setting the threshold at one, two, or three times the standard deviation. In this example, the threshold is plotted directly onto the graph in the form of control limit lines. When a measurement crosses the control limit lines—as do the three elevated measurements—further investigation must occur. The reasons why a measurement crosses a control limit are, of course, unknown until further investigation occurs. (See Appendix C for instructions on how to create and use control charts for setting thresholds for evaluation and tracking indicator data against thresholds.) This chart is filled out with hypothetical rates and is not based on real data.

Source: Adapted from a graph developed by Linda Owen, Quality Assurance Specialist; Judith Quirt, Coordinator, Infection Control Program; Carl Weston, MD, Vice-President, Medical Affairs; and Mary Zimmerman, Director, Quality Resources from Meriter Hospital, Inc, Madison, WI, 1990. Used with permission.

STEP 6 Collect and Organize Data

For each indicator, data must be collected and organized so that those responsible can apply thresholds and determine when further evaluation must occur. To collect and organize data, staff members need to determine the following for each indicator:

- The appropriateness of sampling;

- The frequency of data collection; and

- The process for comparing cumulative data with the thresholds for evaluation.

This step also involves the initial testing of data sources and data-collection method determined as part of developing the indicators (Step 4). There may well be problems in the data collection plan that must be worked out. The data sources and collection methodology should be evaluated for accuracy and reliability; also, the validity of the threshold(s) for evaluation should be reevaluated.

Sampling

For each indicator, staff members should decide whether sampling is appropriate for data collection. Sampling (ie, reviewing only a percentage of pertinent cases/medical records) is generally inappropriate for sentinel-event indicators that address infrequent but serious occurrences (eg, maternal death). In contrast, monitoring that focuses on high-volume procedures may necessarily involve only a sample of patients owing to time and resource limitations.

Frequency of collection

The frequency with which data are collected and tabulated should be based on the risk involved in the care, the frequency with which the aspect of care is performed, and the extent to which the aspect of care has been demonstrated to be problem free. It is important that the organization have a systematic plan for collecting data on a prearranged, ongoing basis.

Comparing data with thresholds

As data are tabulated, the cumulative data for each indicator should periodically be compared with its corresponding threshold for evaluation. This comparison is used to determine whether further evaluation must occur. If thresholds are not breached, routine monitoring is still continued, and the results are again compared to thresholds at the end of the next monitoring period.

If no opportunities for improvement are found after sufficient time elapses (eg, six months, one year), the choice of important aspects of care or service, the indicators, their thresholds for evaluation, and the data-collection methods should be reevaluated to determine their utility in assessing the aspects of care or service addressed by the indicator. Changes might be made in the indicator, threshold, and/or data-collection method to make them more effective in identifying opportunities for improvement. (For more on how to make such changes see the Joint Commission publication *Primer on Indicator Development and Application: Measuring Quality in Health Care.*)

OTHER QUALITY-RELATED FEEDBACK CAN TRIGGER EVALUATION

Leaders and others in the organization must establish channels by which they receive feedback that is not part of ongoing monitoring, but that is related to the quality of care and service. This feedback may come from surveys, comments, suggestions, and complaints of staff, patients, patients' families, and others who use the organization's services. This aspect of data-collection (which is not included in the current description of the monitoring and evaluation process) recognizes that information from sources outside ongoing monitoring can and should be used to trigger further evaluation and efforts to improve.

Data collection is the one step in monitoring and evaluation that normally requires some sort of form, both to collect data and to organize what has been collected. There are many possible variations of data collection/organization forms, and each health care organization should be creative in adapting or creating its own. Data collection forms should be simple to use, requiring the least possible amount of writing to complete them. Adding the code number of the practitioner, shift involved, and other data for each occurrence recorded can be helpful in discerning patterns of care should a focused evaluation of the data (Step 7) be undertaken. Once data are collected, data organization forms can aid in data aggregation to help ensure clarity and ease of understanding.

Figure 6.A. shows a format for describing the data collection plan for given indicators. (Also see 4.R. through 4.W.; in particular, Figures 4.U. through 4.W. are forms to help plan data collection strategies as part of indicator development. Figure 4.E. is a checklist to assess the adequacy of data collection plans.)

Figure 6.B. is a form to help identify and limit the use of unapproved abbreviations in data sources such as the medical record.

Aspects of care selected for monitoring and evaluation may be listed on calendars that show when data are to be collected and/or compared to thresholds for evaluation (Figures 6.C. through 6.E.).

Figures 6.F. through 6.V. show a host of forms for collecting indicator data. Despite the subtle differences, each form fulfills a similar purpose: recording whether a given patient, occurrence, procedure, or other factor met the indicator. Different rating scales and ways to show when or where the indicator event occurred are represented.

For some data-collection formats, the person collecting data may only need to check a "yes" column if the indicator is met or a "no" column if it is not. Figures 6.F. and 6.G. allow collection of data for many patients on one form, are easy to fill out manually, and can be used to capture information on rate-based indicators. These forms also make it easy to express cumulative results as a percentage, and to compare that percentage with the threshold for evaluation.

One of the forms for reporting data generated by the Joint Commission's recommended clinical indicators appears as Figure 6.R. Incident reports (Figures 6.U. and 6.V.) round out these data collection forms.

Once data have been collected, they must be aggregated, organized, and compared with the threshold for evaluation. Data can be highlighted to show whether they meet the threshold for evaluation (Figures 6.W. and 6.X.). A calendar-type format facilitates reporting of monthly or quarterly occurence levels (Figure 6.Y.). Data can be presented so as to show percentage of improvement or decline since previous monitoring periods (Figure 6.Z.).

For rate-based indicators, it is necessary when reporting an indicator's rate of occurrence to list the total number of patients for whom the event could have occurred (that is, the number of patients who have the condition, disease, or procedure the indicator is monitoring). For example, a report on the rate at which cerebrovascular accident patients develop congestive heart failure (ie, the numerator of the indicator occurrence rate) should include the total number of cerebrovascular accident patients (ie, the denominator of the occurrence rate).

Other reporting formats appear as Figures 6.AA. through 6.DD. As Figure 6.EE. indicates, data can also be organized graphically (see Chapter 7 for more examples of graphic presentation of data). Figure 6.FF. is a form to tabulate results of a satisfaction survey.

A Completed QA/RM Management Profile Analysis

Quality Assurance/ Risk Management Activity	Results Reported to	Minutes Filed in	Primary Data Sources	QA Specialist Support Personnel (Title/Department)	Clerical Support Personnel (Title/Department)
Dept monitoring & evaluation (M&E)	Each medical (med) department (dept) Quality assurance committee (QA comm) Med staff executive comm (exec comm) Trustees	Med staff office Administration (admin)	Med record (rec)	QA dept	Comm assistant
Nursing M&E	QA comm Each nursing unit Associate (assoc) administrator of patient (pt) care services	Nursing dept Assoc administrator's office	Med rec	Coordinator of policies & procedures Nursing dept	Nursing dept clerical staff
M&E of other depts	Med staff advisory comm	Each dept Med staff office	Departmental recs Med rec	Staff personnel with assistance of QA dept	QA dept
Utilization review	QA comm Exec comm Trustees, all med depts as appropriate	Med staff office Admin	Med rec	QA dept	QA dept Admin
Surgical case review (includes specimen and nonspecimen surgeries)	Surgery (surg) dept Obstetrics/ Gynecology (OB/ GYN) dept, all med depts as appropriate	Med staff office	Med rec	Med staff secretaries (secys)	Med staff secys
Blood utilization	Surg dept, all med depts as appropriate	Laboratory (lab) Med staff office	Blood bank statistics	Blood bank personnel	Lab secys
Antibiotic utilization	Pharmacy (pharm) & therapeutics comm Exec comm, all med depts as appropriate	Pharm dept Med staff office	Pharm rec Med rec	Pharm personnel	Pharm secys

(continued)

A Completed QA/RM Management Profile Analysis (continued)

Quality Assurance/ Risk Management Activity	Results Reported to	Minutes Filed in	Primary Data Sources	QA Specialist Support Personnel (Title/Department)	Clerical Support Personnel (Title/Department)
Pharmacy and therapeutics	Exec comm, all med depts as appropriate	Med staff office	Med rec	QA dept on routine drug audits Pharm	Pharm secys
Medical record review	Med rec comm Accreditation comm Exec comm, all med depts as appropriate	Med staff office	Med rec	Med rec dept Med staff (random review)	Med rec dept
Mortality review	All med staff depts	Med staff office	Med rec	Med staff	Med staff secys
Perinatal morbidity & mortality	OB/GYN dept	Med staff office	Admitting log Med rec	Med rec dept	Med rec dept
Infection control	Exec comm, all med depts as appropriate	Med staff office	Med rec	Infection control nurse in nursing dept	Nursing dept
Safety	Risk management (RM) comm Assoc administrator of employee relations, all med depts as appropriate	Admin Safety officer	Incident reports	Safety officer	Education (ed) & training dept secy
Risk management	RM comm, all med depts as appropriate	RM administrator's office	Incident reports Safety reports	RM administrator's secy	RM administrator's secy
Ombudsman program	CEO	None	Pt & family complaints	Pt representative	Administrative secys
Tumor board	Exec comm Continuing med ed (CME) comm	Med staff office	Med rec	Tumor secy/med rec dept	Med rec dept
Discharge planning	Assoc administrator of professional services	None	Med rec	Social service	Social service
Accreditation	Exec comm	Med staff office	Reports of dept heads & med staff	Med staff secys	Med staff secys
Credentials	Exec comm	Med staff office	Physicians' files Requests of physicians	Med staff secys	Med staff secys
Continuing medical education	Exec comm	Med staff office	Audit reports	Coordinator of CME	Coordinator of CME
Inservice training program	Assoc administrator of employee relations	Ed & training dept	Employee rec Sign-in sheets	Ed & training secy	Ed & training secy
Orientation program	Assoc administrator of employee relations	Ed & training dept	Employee rec Sign-in sheets	Ed & training secy	Ed & training secy
Employee performance reviews	Assoc administrator of employee relations	Personnel dept Nursing dept	Supervisor's form Nursing dept	Individual hospital depts	Individual hospital depts

Figure 6.A. *An overview of data collection strategies for many aspects of quality assurance and risk management.*
Source: *Adapted from Stearns G, Fox LA: Assessing quality assurance and risk management activities: A profile analysis. QRB Special Edition, spring 1980, pp 23-24.*

Acronyms & Abbreviations

_____DEPARTMENT

ABBREVIATIONS FOUND	ON APPROVED LIST YES NO	CATEGORY OF PERSON COMPLETING REQUISITION RN, WC, OTHER (IDENTIFY)	DATE OF REQUISITION	PATIENT NAME	ADMISSION DATE	COMMENTS (WHAT PROBLEMS DID IT CAUSE)	CATEGORY RESPONSIBLE FOR ABBREVIATION, RN, PHYSICIAN, WC, OTHER (IDENTIFY)

FIGURE 6.B. A bewildering array of unapproved acronyms and abbreviations can often cause problems in data collection. This tool is designed to collect instances of unapproved abbreviations in data sources, to help limit the use of abbreviations to those approved, and to update the list of approved abbreviations.
SOURCE: _Adapted from Q.A. Guide: Appropriateness in Patient Care Services. Reston, VA: American College of Radiology, 1983, p 1._

Monitoring and Evaluation Calendar

DEPARTMENT: Diagnostic Radiology   YEAR: 1992

FREQUENCY	ASPECT OF CARE	JAN	FEB	MAR	APR	MAY	JUN	JUL	AUG	SEP	OCT	NOV	DEC
M O N T H L Y	1. Film retakes				30	30	30	30	30	30			
	2. X-rays	15	15	15	15	15	15						
	3. Pregnancy identification procedures						30	30	30	30	30	30	30
B I M O N T H L Y	1. Sequencing of studies	1		1		1		1		1		1	
	2. Clinical detail on study requests								15		15		15
	3. Breast cancer diagnosis accuracy				30		30		30		30		30
Q U A R T E R L Y	1. 24-hour staffing			1			1			1			1
	2. Informed consent			15			15						

FIGURE 6.C. *A monitoring and evaluation calendar for data organization. Dates in each month denote when data are to be compiled and compared with thresholds for evaluation.*

Monitoring and Evaluation Plan

DEPARTMENT   MONTH

Monitoring and Evaluation Functions	J Due/Met	F Due/Met	M Due/Met	A Due/Met	M Due/Met	J Due/Met	J Due/Met	A Due/Met	S Due/Met	O Due/Met	N Due/Met	D Due/Met
Medical Records												
Pharmacy and Therapeutics Drug Usage Evaluation												
Blood Usage Review												
Surgical Case Review												
Utilization Review												
Risk Management												
Infection Control												
Other (Safety, ICU)												
Departmental Indicators												
Generic Occurrence Screens												
Other												
x = Due √ = Met												

FIGURE 6.D. *Used to demonstrate when medical staff departments should report items at their monthly meetings, this calendar addresses many functions of quality assurance and risk management, including the monitoring schedule of specific indicators. Vertical columns allow documenting the completion of scheduled tasks.*
SOURCE: *Adapted from Edgar Blount, MD, consultant, Quality Healthcare Resources (QHR), Inc, a not-for-profit consulting subsidiary of the Joint Commission, Oakbrook Terrace, IL.*

Monitoring and Evaluation Data Collection and Tabulation Calendar

Key: * = Collect
0 = Tabulation comparison to thresholds

SAFETY COMMITTEE	JAN	FEB	MAR	APR	MAY	JUN	JUL	AUG	SEP	OCT	NOV	DEC
Patient falls	*0	*	*	*0	*	*	*0	*	*	*0	*	*
Medication variances	*	*0	*	*	*0	*	*	*0	*	*	*0	*
Nosocomial infections	*	*	*0	*	*	*0	*	*	*0	*	*	*0
Patient satisfaction	*	*	*0	*	*	*0	*	*	*0	*	*	*0
ASPECTS OF CARE:												
Oxygenation	*0	*0							*0	*0		
Comfort	*0	*0									*0	*0
Nutrition			*0	*0							*0	*0
Activity			*0	*0								
Management of health					*0	*0						
Coping					*0	*0						
Elimination							*0	*0				
Protection							*0	*0				
Growth and development									*0	*0		

FIGURE 6.E. *Form allows scheduling and documenting both data collection and comparison to thresholds for evaluation.*
SOURCE: *Robert Wood Johnson University Hospital, New Brunswick, NJ. Used with permission.*

Sample Data Collection Tool

MONTH/YEAR: _____

IMPORTANT ASPECT OF CARE:

Patient Number	Staff Number	Shift/ Date	Indicator 1		Indicator 2		Indicator 3		Indicator 4		Remarks
			Yes	No	Yes	No	Yes	No	Yes	No	
Total											
Percentage of the total sample											
Threshold for evaluation											
Evaluation of data required?											
Percentage for previous monitoring period											
Percent improvement											

FIGURE 6.F. *Data collection form that allows data collection for multiple indicators and multiple patients. Columns ask for the staff member in charge of caring for the patient, shift, and date. The form also facilitates translating collected data into a rate of occurrence and comparing that percentage to the threshold for evaluation. Many variations upon this form are possible; for example, vertical columns can be added on the left asking for the age and sex of the patient, nurse number, or other information. The indicators might be printed (for the data collector to refer to) in the upper left corner.*
SOURCE: *Shirley Noah, RN, consultant, Quality Healthcare Resources, Inc, a not-for-profit subsidiary of the Joint Commission, Oakbrook Terrace, IL.*

Monitoring and Evaluation Worksheet—Dental

I. Facility Identification

Activity or Provider Reviewed *(Identify provider by number)*		Reviewed by *(Identify reviewer by number)*		Date
Dental QA/RM committee review	Date	SGD Review *(Optional)*		Date

II. Evaluation Comments

III. Patient Identification
(1 through 10 indicate individual patient records; S indicates summary of 1-10.)

	1	2	3	4	5	6	7	8	9	10	S
Patient Initials											
Family Member Prefix											
Social Security Number											

IV. Aspects of Care and Indicators

1. Aspect of Care: Biopsies

☐ A. *Indicator:* Biopsy submitted properly:
  (1) Proper preparation of specimens for shipment IAW AFR 162-1.
  (2) Returned SF 515 indicates adequate specimen submitted.

☐ B. *Indicator:* Biopsy results are documented:
  (1) Completed SF 515 is included in the dental record.
  (2) Pertinent information is transcribed from completed SF 515 to SF 603/603A. These items include:

    a. Date pathology report returned.
    b. Case accession number.
    c. Facility providing diagnosis.
    d. Diagnosis.
    e. Patient notification *(if appropriate).*
    f. Required follow-up.

V. Thresholds
(Key: Y = Yes   N = No   O = Not Applicable)

Threshold											
10%											
10%											
10%											
10%											

	1	2	3	4	5	6	7	8	9	10	S

Key: Y = Yes   N = No   O = Not Applicable

Threshold	1	2	3	4	5	6	7	8	9	10	S

2. Aspect of Care: Cast Restorations

☐ A. *Indicator:* Treatment is properly planned:
  (1) Radiographs include the apical area(s) of the teeth and are evaluated prior to preparation of the teeth.

10%											

☐ B. *Indicator:* Interim restorations are placed.
  (1) Protective provisional restorations are placed on prepared teeth while definitive restoration is being fabricated.

10%											

Figure 6.G. *The first page of a data collection form for dental care monitoring and evaluation.*
Source: *United States Air Force Dental Service, HQ USAF/SGD, Bolling AFB, DC. Implementation date: Aug 1988.*

Checklist Style of Patient Classification

Instructions:

Check (✔) applicable statement for each classification in the appropriate patient column. Add total points to place patient in a category.

Total Points	Category
0-11	I
12-21	II
22+-30	III
30+-	IV

PATIENT:

AGE:

ROOM:

			D A T E Acuity Level												
EATING	Self-Care	1													
	Help Setting Up	2													
	Feed—Tube Feed	3													
	Feed with Problem Frequent Tube Feedings	4													
GROOM	Self-Bed Bath	1													
	Complete Care	2													
	Complete Care Problems	3													
EXCRET	Self-Care	1													
	Needs Help	2													
	Needs Frequent Help	3													
	Incontinent	4													
ACTIVITY	Ambulatory	1													
	Ambulatory with Help	2													
	Ambulatory or Turn with 2	3													
	Frequently Ambulatory with Help Complicating Apparatus	4													
BEHAVIOR	Alert—Oriented	1													
	Mildly Confused	2													
	Restraints—Confused	3													
	Demanding/Psychotic	4													
TEACHING	Routine	1													
	Reinforcement	2													
	New Detailed Emotional Support	3													
	Communication Barrier	4													
TREATMENT	Routine Bedside Equipment	1													
	Cath Care Sitz—Moist Comp	2													
	Traction Decubitus Care	3													
	Frequent Suction—Tubes Wound Irrigation (Several)	4													
MEDICATION	Routine	1													
	Topical Ointments: Pre-Post OP/KVO IVs	2													
	8 IV/IVPB Many Meds PO	3													
	Frequent PRNs & IVPB Combination of Meds	4													
	Transfusion/TPN															
	Total Patient Acuity															

FIGURE 6.H. *Data collection checklist to measure patients' acuity level over time as it relates to activities for daily living and other factors. The form includes a point scale in the upper left-hand corner for classifying each patient.*
SOURCE: *Lewis EN, Carini PV:* Nursing Staffing and Patient Classification: Strategies for Success. *Rockville, MD: Aspen Publishers, 1984.*

Wristband Identification Error Reporting Worksheet

Section One. Patients with Wristband I.D. Errors:		COLUMN:	A Wristband Absent	B Wristband From Another Patient	C Patient Wearing More Than One Wristband	D Partially Missing I.D. Information	E Partially Erroneous I.D. Information	F Illegible I.D. Information
Patient Name	I.D. Number	Date						
1.								
2.								
3.								
4.								
5.								
6.								
7.								
8.								
9.								
10.								
11.								
12.								
13.								
14.								
15.								
16.								
17.								
18.								
19.								
20.								

Item G:

Total Number of Patients with
I.D. Errors this Page: _____

Totals: ____ ____ ____ ____ ____ ____
A   B   C   D   E   F

Section Two.

Number of Patients Drawn (and Checked for Wristband I.D. Adequacy) Each Day During the
Q-Probes Monitoring Period:

Date	No.	Date	No.	Date	No.	Date	No.
___/___/___ : ___		___/___/___ : ___		___/___/___ : ___		___/___/___ : ___	
___/___/___ : ___		___/___/___ : ___		___/___/___ : ___		___/___/___ : ___	
___/___/___ : ___		___/___/___ : ___		___/___/___ : ___		___/___/___ : ___	
___/___/___ : ___		___/___/___ : ___		___/___/___ : ___		___/___/___ : ___	
___/___/___ : ___		___/___/___ : ___		___/___/___ : ___		___/___/___ : ___	
___/___/___ : ___		___/___/___ : ___		___/___/___ : ___		___/___/___ : ___	
___/___/___ : ___		___/___/___ : ___		___/___/___ : ___		___/___/___ : ___	
___/___/___ : ___		___/___/___ : ___		___/___/___ : ___			

Section Two: Total _____

FIGURE 6.I. Data collection form for patient ''ID'' wristband error.
SOURCE: College of American Pathologists, Northfield, IL, 1990. Used with permission.

Community Treatment Program Quality Assurance Worksheet													
					Date _____								
						CHARTS EXAMINED							
INDICATORS	YES	NO	N/A	COMMENTS									

FIGURE 6.J. *Another layout to show that a particular indicator was met for multiple patients.*
SOURCE: *Mackay C, with the assistance of Davis LL: Community treatment program quality assurance plan.* Q Resource Monitor *special supplement, 3(4):25, Jul/Aug 1987.*

Data Collection Worksheet

MR# _____   Attending _____   Reviewed By _____

Age _____   Sex _____

Diagnosis:

	Check the appropriate indication for transfusion under components					
Indicator	Threshold for Evaluation	Met		Met after Committee Review		Action
		Y	N	Y	N	

FIGURE 6.K. *Data collection worksheet with columns asking whether transfusions were justified.* **SOURCE:** *Gail Bronswick, manager, professional services, Quality Healthcare Resources, Inc, a not-for-profit subsidiary of the Joint Commission, Oakbrook Terrace, IL.*

The Ervin Quality Assessment Measurement Instrument

INDICATOR	MET	NOT MET	IF MET, INDICATE THE EXTENT TO WHICH CRITERION WAS MET*					COMMENTS
			1	2	3	4	5	
Assessment								
Data were documented to support identified problems								
All problems that were implied from the data base were identified								
Data base was updated continuously								
Status of problems was updated continuously								
Planning								
Nursing care plan was coordinated with goals of other care providers, as appropriate								
Spacing of home visits was based on care plan								
The plan of care was altered based on changing family needs								
Implementation								
Nursing interventions were executed for the identified problems								
The family was involved in implementation of the nursing care plan								
Revisits were done or attempted as planned								
Evaluation								
Patient outcomes or progress with plan of care was stated								
Follow-up was complete on all problems								
The plan of care was evaluated with client or family								
The plan of care was revised to reflect the results of the evaluation, if appropriate								

*1 = slightly   2 = somewhat   3 = about half   4 = almost totally   5 = totally

FIGURE 6.L. *Form not only requires the data collector to show whether the indicator event was present, but also to record the extent to which this was the case.*
SOURCE: *Ervin NE, Chen SC, Upshaw H: Development of a public health nursing quality assessment measure. QRB 15(5): 141, May 1989.*

Guidelines—Nursing Documentation Review

Nursing Practice Standards Assessment

Patient Name _____ Medical History # _____ Admit Date _____ Review Date _____

Criterion/Applicability	Special Instructions	Response
1.4 Each narrative note written by an RN is referenced to a problem (problem name) on the master problem list or patient care plan. /All	Exception: temporary problems; referenced in the note but does not appear on problem list or care plan. Check all the notes for the most recent complete 24-hour period in the progress record. Each RN note must meet criterion or enter NO.	YES NO NA
1.5 Each narrative note written by the RN contains: a. subjective information or ☐ objective information b. assessment ☐ c. plan ☐ /All	Review a note written by an RN during the most recent 24 hours. Must have a ✔ in each box to rate YES. If there is no note written by an RN mark NA*.	YES NO NA*
1.6 There is documentation of the implementation of nursing orders (plans). /All	Refer to the care plan (Kardex), select the one most recent nursing order, then look for evidence that the order was carried out. Evidence of plan implementation may be found on patient record, flow sheets, parenteral fluid sheets or medication record, or any other legitimate chart form. A code of NA* indicates no plans documented.	YES NO NA*
1.7 There is documentation of the evaluation of patient's response to nursing orders. /All	Refer to care plan/Kardex for short- or long-term goal. Look for evidence indicative of patient's response to nursing interventions and/or progress or lack of progress toward goal most recent 48 hours. A code of NA* indicates no goals or plans documented.	YES NO NA*
1.8 Progress notes written by auxiliary personnel are cosigned by an RN. /All	Review notes written in most recent 48 hours.	YES NO NA
	TOTALS	YES NO NA NA*

Figure 6.M. *As on this form, many data collection forms include instructions for data collection, exceptions, definitions, or hints on the interpretation of patient records. This figure is the first page of a multi-page form.*
Source: *Group Health Cooperative of Puget Sound, Seattle. Used with permission.*

Two Formats for Recording Indicator Data for Multiple Hospitals

Month, Year: _____

Group	Indicators	Hospitals																				Total
		1	2	3	4	5	6	7	8	9	10	11	12	13	14	15	16	17	18	19	20	
Medical Staff, Nursing Service, & Other Ancillary Services																						

Month, Year: _____

Hospital	Indicators									

Figure 6.N. Two possible formats to organize and display indicator data on multiple health care organizations. These formats would be appropriate for a multifacility chain.

Questionnaire on Knowledge of Patients with Myocardial Infarction

PATIENT QUESTIONS	FACTORS FROM THE CHART	PATIENT RESPONSES CORRECT/INCORRECT
1. What did the tests show was wrong with you?	Type of MI	
2. What type of physical activities are you allowed to do now?	Rehab level or MD activity order	
3. Which medications are you taking now and what are they for? (List the name of the pill, if you know it, otherwise describe the way it looks or what it does.)	List the meds from the med sheet	
4. What is a heart attack?	Definition from printed information given to patient	
5. What past or present illnesses or life-styles do you feel have caused your present illness?	Risk factors	
6. How long do you think you will be in the hospital?	Name of physician _____ Time told by physician _____	
7. What will your treatment be for this illness between now and the time you go home?	Rehabilitation program?; classes?; rest?	
8. After you go home from the hospital, will you need to change your daily activities? (example—job, hobbies, etc)	On special diet?; any restrictions that you know of?	
9. Could this ever happen to you again?		
10. What questions do you have that were not answered during your stay in this unit?		

Did the patient get any printed information? How many days ago?

Teaching documented?

FIGURE 6.O. *Questionnaire/data collection form probes the knowledge of patients with myocardial infarction concerning their own condition and self-care regimen. Such a form is one way to measure how well patient education has been carried out.*
SOURCE: *St Michael Hospital, Milwaukee, Copyright 1982. Used with permission.*

Patient Teaching Checklist Newborn Education Record

PLACE A DATE AND YOUR INITIALS IN THE APPROPRIATE BOXES TO DESIGNATE PATIENT TEACHING PERFORMED

Topics Presented	Initial Instruction	Patient Verbalizes	Patient Demonstrates	Follow-up Reinforcement	Comments
I. PHYSICAL CARE					
A. Baby Bath					
B. Cord Care					
C. Circumcision Care					
D. Diapering & Dressing					
E. Temperature					
II. ELIMINATION					
A. Urination					
B. Bowel Patterns					
III. FEEDING					
A. Breast					
1. Correct Technique					
2. "Latching On" & Breaking Suction					
3. Alternate Position					
4. Frequency of Feedings					
5. Breast Pump Use					
B. Bottle					
1. Correct Technique					
2. Use & Care of Equipment					
3. Alternate Types of Formula & Preparation					
4. Amount & Frequency of Feedings					
C. Bubbling					
IV. SIGNS & SYMPTOMS OF ILLNESS					
V. INFECTION PREVENTION					
VI. CAR SEAT SAFETY					

PHYSICIAN'S INSTRUCTIONS GIVEN			PATIENT STAMP
R.N. INITIALS & SIGNATURE:	FILMS VIEWED:		
	WRITTEN INFORMATION GIVEN:		
I VERIFY THAT I UNDERSTAND THE ABOVE INFORMATION			
MOTHER'S SIGNATURE			
DISCHARGE NURSE'S SIGNATURE			

FIGURE 6.P. *Form to record whether a patient has been adequately educated about self care (or, in this case, infant care). This form facilitates recording of both whether the patient can verbally describe adequate infant care and whether he or she can demonstrate such care.*
SOURCE: *Central Dupage Hospital, Winfield, IL. Used with permission.*

Film Analysis Report

Date	Exam	Film Size	Initial	Repeat				Scrap
				Motion	Dark	Light	Position	

FIGURE 6.Q. *Form to record data on the frequency and causes of radiology film rejects. An important method for verifying the accuracy of this monitoring is to have a single place to "pitch" rejected films and periodically compare the number of rejects to the number on the film analysis report.*
SOURCE: Q.A. Guide: Appropriateness in Patient Care Services. *Reston, VA: American College of Radiology, 1983, p 19.*

MEDICAL RECORD NUMBER _____   DISCHARGE DATE ___/___/___

Maternal Record

Maternal Medical Record Number: _____

Maternal discharge date: ___/___/___

1) Mother's admission date ___/___/___

2) Admission Time (24 hr) _____

3) Admission source: _____
   1. physician referral
   2. clinic referral
   3. HMO referral
   4. transfer from another hospital
   5. transfer from an SNF
   6. transfer from another health care facility
   7. emergency room
   8. court/law enforcement
   9. information not available

4) Type of admission: _____
   1. emergency
   2. urgent
   3. elective

5) Discharge date: ___/___/___

6) Time of discharge (24 hr): _____

7) Discharge disposition: _____
   01. discharged home
   02. discharged/transferred to another acute care facility
   03. discharged/transferred to a skilled nursing care facility
   04. discharged/transferred to an intermediate care facility
   05. discharged/transferred to another type of facility
   06. discharged/transferred to home under home care services
   07. left against medical advice
   20. expired

8) Mother's date of birth: ___/___/___

9) Zip code of residence _____

10) Race and ethnicity: _____
    A American Indian or Alaskan native
    R Asian or Pacific islander
    B Black
    H Hispanic
    C Caucasion
    O Other
    U Unknown

11) Marital Status: _____
    S single
    M married
    X legally separated
    D divorced
    W widowed
    U unknown

12) Expected principle source of payment: _____
    01 self pay
    02 workmen's compensation
    03 Medicare
    04 Medicaid
    05 maternal and child health
    06 other government payments
    07 Blue Cross
    08 insurance company
    09 HMO
    10 no charge
    11 other
    12 unknown

13) Maternal Principal ICD-9-CM diagnosis at discharge

    _____

(continued)

MEDICAL RECORD NUMBER _____   DISCHARGE DATE ___/___/___

Maternal Record (continued)

14) If other ICD-9-CM diagnoses were present at discharge enter them below.

   _____   _____   _____
   _____   _____   _____
   _____   _____   _____
   _____   _____   _____
   _____   _____   _____

15) Maternal principal ICD-9-CM date and procedure code at discharge:
   ___/___/___   _____

16) Other dates and procedure codes at discharge

date	code	date	code
___/___/___	_____	___/___/___	_____
___/___/___	_____	___/___/___	_____
___/___/___	_____	___/___/___	_____
___/___/___	_____	___/___/___	_____
___/___/___	_____	___/___/___	_____
___/___/___	_____	___/___/___	_____
___/___/___	_____	___/___/___	_____
___/___/___	_____		

Labor and Delivery Section

17a) Gravida: ____   17b) Parity: ____   18) Estimated length of gestation: ____

19) Was onset of labor: ____
   1. spontaneous
   2. induced
   3. indeterminate
   4. no labor

20) Place of delivery: ____
   1. present hosptial
   2. en route to hospital
   3. other

21) Did the patient have a prior history of cesarean section? ____
   1. no
   2. yes

> Answer question 22 if the patient had a history of prior cesarean section
> 22) Was a vaginal birth attempted: ____
>   1. no
>   2. yes

23) Date of delivery: ___/___/___   24) Time of delivery (24 hr): ____

25) Fetal heartbeat present at admission: ____
   1. no
   2. yes
   3. not documented

26) Number of liveborn infants this delivery: ____

27) Was there a stillbirth: ____
   1. no
   2. yes

(continued)

MEDICAL RECORD NUMBER _____   DISCHARGE DATE ____/____/____

Maternal Record (continued)

Complete this section only for stillbirths

28) Number of stillborn infants: _____

29) Weight scale used: _____
   1. lbs/oz
   2. grams

30) Stillborn infant weights (enter grams as a whole number, enter lbs/oz as lb-oz example: 07-03 for 7 lbs, 3 oz or 2500 for 2500 grams)

   a _____   b _____   c _____   d _____   e _____   f _____

Laboratory Section:

31) Lowest predelivery Hgb: _____ gm

32) Lowest postdelivery Hgb: _____ gm

33) Lowest predelivery Hct: _____ %

34) Lowest postdelivery Hct: _____ %

35) Did the mother receive an intra- and/or postpartum red blood cell transfusion: _____
   1. no
   2. yes

Optional data

36) Attending physician ID: _____

37) Operating physician ID: _____

38) Abstractor number: _____

39) Data entry number: _____

FIGURE 6.R. The first (maternal) part of the data collection tool for the Joint Commission's recommended indicators.

Lung Cancer FNAC Diagnostic Performance

INSTRUCTIONS TO PARTICIPANTS

Part 1: Fine Needle Aspiration Cytology (FNAC)-Histologic Tissue Diagnosis Correlation

1. In reviewing your FNAC records, it will help to group the reports into three separate categories: satisfactory, unsatisfactory and technically inadequate FNACs. You will be comparing only the diagnoses from satisfactory FNACs with corresponding histologic tissue diagnoses.

2. Obtain patient FNAC case number and diagnosis for each satisfactory lung FNAC performed within the study time period. Record the FNAC case number and diagnosis on the appropriate FNAC worksheet:
   - Diagnosis of malignancy by FNAC (use Worksheet 1)
   - Benign, no diagnosis of malignancy by FNAC (use Worksheet 2)

   You may photocopy the worksheets if additional space is needed.

3. Next, obtain surgical pathology reports for each satisfactory FNAC and list the diagnosis next to the corresponding FNAC diagnosis on the appropriate worksheet. For those with histologic correlation available, compare the diagnoses for any concordance/discordance between diagnoses of benign and malignant. Discordance will most likely result from interpretation or sampling differences between the two techniques and will require a review of slides (interpretation discrepancy) and/or clinical information (sampling discrepancy). If, after thorough review discordance still exists, consultation with the clinician will be necessary to correlate clinical outcome.

Note: For this analysis, do not consider differences in diagnoses by tissue type (eg. carcinoma vs. lymphoma) or histologic tumor subtyping (eg. small cell vs. non-small cell carcinoma). These will be enumerated separately in Part 3.

4. Match corresponding histologic tissue diagnoses to the descriptors A-H defined on the FNAC Tally Sheet (summarized below). Tabulate totals on the FNAC Tally Sheet for your records, then transcribe descriptor category totals to FNAC input Form 1A. For descriptor category "Other" (Descriptor I), use FNAC input Form 2.

Note: Descriptor is used only for histology-correlated FNACs that do not fit the usual descriptor categories A-H (for example, pretherapeutic FNAC diagnosis of malignancy followed by a negative tissue resection due to complete pathologic remission by chemotherapy or radiotherapy).

FNAC Category	Corresponding Descriptors
Malignancy diagnosed by FNAC (positive or suspicious/suggestive of cancer)	A-D
Benign FNAC diagnoses (negative, malignancy not diagnosed)	E-H
Other	I

(continued)

Lung Cancer FNAC Diagnostic Performance (continued)

Part 2: Patient Management Categories

5. For each FNAC occurrence tabulated as Descriptor D (false positive FNAC) and Descriptor F (false negative FNAC), categorize the effect in patient management using the following scheme:

- Patient management unaffected
- Patient management minimally affected (such that effect on patient outcome could be classified as temporary minor, temporary major, or permanent minor).

- Patient management greatly affected (such that effect on patient outcome could be classified as permanent significant, permanent major, permanent grave, or death).

Tabulate totals on FNAC input Form 1A. The three management categories must add up to the total for each descriptor.

Part 3: Discordance in Histologic Tissue Typing of Malignancy

6. The correlation of FNAC and histologic tissue diagnoses for Descriptors A thru I is restricted to diagnoses of malignancy of benignancy. Occassionally, discrepancies in the histologic tissue typing of malignancy may arise. These are not considered as discordance on the FNAC Tally Sheet. Should these discrepancies of malignant diagnoses by tissue typing (carcinoma versus lymphoma) or tumor subtyping (small cell versus non-small cell carcinoma) arise, enumerate totals under Part 3 on Input Form 1A (Descriptors J, K, and L).

Part 4: Additional Data

7. In the appropriate sections of FNAC Input Form 1B, tabulate the number of occurrences of the following:

- the number of satisfactory lung FNAC cases with histologic correlation available (X) (This number should equal the sum of Descriptors A-L or a maximum of 50 cases.)

- the number of lung FNACs found unsatisfactory for evaluation in 1989 (Y)

- the number of lung FNACs found technically inadequate for evaluation in 1989 (Z)

- the total number of lung FNACs accessioned within the study period (1989) with and without histologic correlation available, including aspirates deemed unsatisfactory or technically inadequate for evaluation.

- the number of pathologists interpreting lung FNACs in your institution

8. Check off the person(s) routinely performing the lung aspiration procedures in your institution on FNAC Input Form 1B.

(continued)

Lung Cancer FNAC Diagnostic Performance (continued)

LUNG CANCER FNAC TALLY SHEET

Occurrences	Descr.	Initial FNAC Diagnosis	Histologic Tissue Diagnosis	Review FNAC/ Tissue	Explanation
	A	True positive FNAC	True positive biopsy	No need	Diagnosis of same malignancy by both methods.
	B	True positive FNAC	False negative biopsy (sampling)	Yes	Tissue biopsy sampling discrepancy. Clinical review confirms FNAC result.
	C	True positive FNAC	False negative biopsy (Interpretation)	Yes	Tissue biopsy interpretation discrepancy. Slide review confirms FNAC result.
	D	False positive FNAC (interpretation)	True negative biopsy	Yes	Erroneous initial FNAC Interpretation. Slide review does not confirm FNAC result.
	E	False negative FNAC (sampling)	True positive biopsy	Yes	FNAC sampling discrepancy. Clinical review confirms positive tissue diagnosis.
	F	False negative FNAC (interpretation)	True positive biopsy	Yes	Erroneous Initial FNAC Interpretation. Slide review confirms positive tissue biopsy result.
	G	True negative FNAC	False positive biopsy (interpretation)	Yes	Tissue biopsy interpretation discrepancy. Slide review confirms negative FNAC result.
	H	True negative FNAC	True negative biopsy	No need	No diagnosis of malignancy by either method.
	I	Other (specify on Input Form 2)	Other (specify on Input Form 2)	Yes	Other explanation for mismatch not identified above. Specify (eg, positive FNAC with negative tissue biopsy following chemotherapy).

positive = malignancy   *biopsy = histologic tissue diagnosis on any excised tissue or postmortem*
negative = no malignancy

(continued)

Lung Cancer FNAC Diagnostic Performance (continued)

MALIGNANCY DIAGNOSED BY FNAC

FNAC Case #	FNAC Diagnosis	Histology Case #	Tissue Diagnosis	Descriptor Category (A, B, C, or D)

MALIGNANCY NOT DIAGNOSED BY FNAC

FNAC Case #	FNAC Diagnosis	Histology Case #	Tissue Diagnosis	Descriptor Category (E, F, G, or H)

(continued)

Lung Cancer FNAC Diagnostic Performance (continued)

PART 1: FNAC-HISTOLOGIC TISSUE DIAGNOSIS CORRELATION

PART 2: MANAGEMENT CATEGORIES

Descriptor   Occurrences

A
B
C
D
E
F
G
H
I

Descriptor	Management Category	Occurrences
D (false positive FNAC)	unaffected minimally affected greatly affected	
F (false negative FNAC)	unaffected minimally affected greatly affected	

(specify on Input Form 2)

PART 3: DISCORDANCE IN HISTOLOGIC TISSUE TYPING OF MALIGNANCY

Descriptor	Discordance	Occurrences
J	Carcinoma versus Lymphoma	
K	Small Cell versus Non-Small Cell Carcinoma	
L	Other Histologic Discordance	

PART 4: ADDITIONAL DATA

Total number of satisfactory FNACs with histologic correlation available   (X) ⬚ (total A thru L)

Total number of FNACs unsatisfactory for evaluation   (Y) ⬚

Total number of FNACs technically inadequate for evaluation   (Z) ⬚

Total FNACs accessioned during study period   ⬚

Total number of pathologists interpreting FNACs in your institution   ⬚

Who routinely performs lung FNAC procedures in your institution:
☐ 1) pathologists
☐ 2) non-pathologists
☐ 3) both

(continued)

Lung Cancer FNAC Diagnostic Performance (continued)

Descriptor I • Other*

Occurrences	Initial FNAC Diagnosis	Histologic Tissue Diagnosis	Review	Explanation

Enumerate and specify each Descriptor I occurrence

* *Use only for histology-correlated FNAC that do not fit into descripter categories A–H. Do not use for a listing of unsatisfactory FNAC or FNAC with no histologic correlation.*

FIGURE 6.S. *Multipage data collection tool comparing initial pathology diagnosis of lung cancer with corresponding histologic tissue diagnosis. The objective of monitoring is to evlauate performance of fine needle aspiration cytology (FNAC) to help assess the effect of FNAC discordant interpretation of malignancy on patient management.*
Source: *College of American Pathologists, Northfield, IL, 1990. Used with permission.*

Emergency Center

Addressograph:
Pt #
Name
DOB

Hospital
[A] [B] [C] [D] [E] [F] [G] [H] [I] [J] [K] [L] [M]
[N] [O] [P] [Q] [R] [S] [T] [U] [V] [W] [X] [Y] [Z]

PATIENT INCIDENT OCCURRENCE REPORT

All information provided on this form including any appended materials and data, is privileged and confidential, and is furnished as a report to the Quality Assurance Committee of the Medical Staff for the purpose of improving the quality of patient care, and to University Legal Counsel as communication prepared in the event of litigation.

GENERAL INFORMATION

[ ] Inpatient
[ ] Outpatient
[ ] Emergency

Age [0] [1] [2] [3] [4] [5] [6] [7] [8] [9]
[10] [20] [30] [40] [50] [60] [70] [80] [90]
Sex [M] [F]

Attending (Inpatient)

Resident

Primary Nurse

Room # [0] [1] [2] [3] [4] [5] [6] [7]
[E] [W] [G] [L] [R]
[ ] Other   [0] [1] [2] [3] [4] [5] [6] [7] [8] [9]
[0] [1] [2] [3] [4] [5] [6] [7] [8] [9]

DATE
JAN FEB MAR APR
MAY JUN JUL AUG
SEP OCT NOV DEC

DAY
[1] [2] [3] [4] [5] [6] [7] [8] [9] [10] [11] [12]
[13] [14] [15] [16] [17] [18] [19] [20] [21] [22] [23] [24]
[25] [26] [27] [28] [29] [30] [31]

Century [19] [20]   Year
[00] [10] [20] [30] [40] [50] [60]
[70] [80] [90] [1] [2] [3] [4]
[5] [6] [7] [8] [9]

TIME [0] [1] [2] [3] [4] [5] [6] [7]
[8] [9] [10] [11] [12] [13] [14] [15]
[16] [17] [18] [19] [20] [21] [22] [23]
MIN [00] [15] [30] [45]

PATIENT CONDITION/ ACTIVITY PRIOR TO INCIDENT OCCURRENCE (Check all that apply)

Physical Problems
[ ] Aphasic
[ ] Bowel/Bladder Problem
[ ] Handicapped
[ ] Hearing Impairment
[ ] Neurological Impairment
[ ] Paralyzed, Complete
[ ] Paralyzed, Partial
[ ] Visual Impairment
[ ] Weak/Faint
[ ] Other
[ ] Unknown

Behavior
[ ] Agitated
[ ] Angry
[ ] Belligerent
[ ] Cooperative
[ ] Normal
[ ] Pleasant
[ ] Uncooperative
[ ] Other
[ ] Unknown

Ordered Activity
[ ] Bedrest with BRP
[ ] BRP with Assist
[ ] BRP w/o Assist
[ ] Strict Bedrest
[ ] Up with Assist
[ ] Up w/o Assist
[ ] Other
[ ] Unknown

Mental Status
[ ] Anxious
[ ] Confused
[ ] Depressed
[ ] Normal
[ ] Retarded
[ ] Senile
[ ] Suicidal
[ ] Other
[ ] Unknown

Induced Conditions
[ ] Anesthetized
[ ] Intoxicated
[ ] Sedated
[ ] Other
[ ] Unknown

Level of Consciousness
[ ] Conscious
[ ] Semiconscious
[ ] Obtunded
[ ] Comatose
[ ] Unknown
[ ] Other

Comments:

LOCATION (Check one)

[ ] BICU [ ] TICU
[ ] CCU [ ] 5WICU
[ ] NICU [ ] Ambulance
[ ] NSU [ ] Bathroom in Hall
[ ] PICU [ ] Cafeteria
[ ] SICU [ ] Cardiac Vascular Lab

[ ] Delivery Room
[ ] Elevator
[ ] Emergency Center
[ ] Hall Corridor
[ ] Helicopter
[ ] Hospital Physical Therapy

[ ] Labor Room
[ ] Laboratory/Pathology
[ ] Lobby
[ ] Nursing Station
[ ] Parking Garage Lot
[ ] Patient Bathroom

[ ] Patient Room
[ ] Pharmacy
[ ] Radiation Therapy
[ ] Radiology
[ ] Recovery Room
[ ] Rusk Physical Therapy

[ ] Same Day Surgery
[ ] Short Stay Center
[ ] Stairwell
[ ] Treatment Room
[ ] Outpatient Clinic
[ ] Other

OP RM STE#: [1] [2] [3] [4] [5] [6] [7] [8] [9]

GENERAL INCIDENT OCCURRENCE

Medication
[ ] Med dose (s) omitted
[ ] Premature or delayed administration
[ ] Dosage incorrect
[ ] Medication incorrect
[ ] Duplication of med order
[ ] Concentration incorrect
[ ] Route incorrect
[ ] Label incorrect
[ ] Wrong patient
[ ] Med administration technique incorrect
[ ] Med given without order
[ ] Defective product packaging
[ ] Count discrepancy of controlled substance
[ ] Other

IV
[ ] Infusion rate incorrect
[ ] Wrong IV solution fluid
[ ] Defective product packaging
[ ] Premature or delayed administration
[ ] IV solution fluid omitted
[ ] Product malfunction
[ ] Incorrect labeling
[ ] IV order discontinued prematurely
[ ] Infiltration
[ ] Line or dressing displaced by patient
[ ] Incompatible additives to fluid
[ ] Wrong Patient
[ ] Other

Procedure
[ ] Omitted/Cancelled
[ ] Incorrectly Performed
[ ] Not ordered
[ ] Wrong Patient
[ ] Improper Equipment
[ ] Error in computing results
[ ] Results Incorrectly Reported
[ ] Improper Patient Preparation
[ ] Lost Specimen
[ ] Lost Results
[ ] Isolation-Related Event
[ ] Incorrect Diet Served
[ ] Patient ID Problems
[ ] Other

Patient Fall
[ ] Ambulating Assisted
[ ] Ambulating Unassisted
[ ] Bed
[ ] Chair
[ ] Using Toilet
[ ] In Shower or Tub
[ ] Wheelchair
[ ] Cart/Stretcher/Exam/OR Table
[ ] Standing
[ ] Transferring Self
[ ] Transferring Assisted
[ ] Other/Cause Unknown

Equipment
[ ] Struck by Equipment
[ ] Caught in or between
[ ] Failure/Mechanical defect
[ ] Improper Use
[ ] Ventilator Problems
[ ] Other

Contributor(s) to Medication/IV Incident:
[ ] Physician(s)
[ ] Nursing staff
[ ] Pharmacy staff
[ ] Other

If applicable, was incorrect med or IV administered? [ ] Yes [ ] No

Blood Product Transfusion Reaction
(Check all that apply)

Signs/symptoms
[ ] pruritis or urticaria
[ ] fever or chills
[ ] dyspnea or chest pain
[ ] hypotension or shock
[ ] bleeding
[ ] Other

Action Taken
[ ] notified MD
[ ] discontinued transfusion
[ ] continued transfusion after
[ ] medication
[ ] notified blood bank
[ ] Other

PATIENT SAFEGUARDS

Restraints [ ] Ordered [ ] Belt [ ] On
[ ] Not Ordered [ ] Vest [ ] Limb [ ] Off

Siderails [ ] All Down
[ ] All Up Other

Call Light [ ] Accessible [ ] Operative
[ ] Not Accessible [ ] Non-Operative

Bed Height [ ] High [ ] Low

NATURE OF INJURY (Check all that apply)

[ ] Swelling
[ ] Hematoma
[ ] Laceration/Cut

[ ] Abrasion/Contusion
[ ] Irritation
[ ] Tenderness-No Identified Injury

[ ] Dehiscence/Evisceration
[ ] Burn/Scald/Blister
[ ] Sprain/Strain

[ ] Fracture Dislocation
[ ] Needle Stick
[ ] New Neurological Deficit

[ ] Drug-Related Injury
[ ] Tissue Loss

SEVERITY OF INJURY (Check one)

[ ] No apparent injury

[ ] Minor (injury is temporary and does not cause further complications)

[ ] Major (injury is serious, or causes considerable discomfort, or requires extended treatment, or life threatening to the patient)

[ ] Death (The patient's death may be directly attributed to the incident)

[ ] Unable to determine (it is impossible to determine the extent of injury)

(continued)

Occurrence Screens–Emergency Center

☐ 1. Patient seen in the Emergency Center and seen (unplanned) in the Emergency Center again within 7 days.

☐ 2. Patient dies in the Emergency Center

☐ 3. Patient refuses treatment, hospitalization or leaves AMA.

☐ 4. Abnormal diagnostic test results returned to the Emergency Center after patient discharge and patient not contacted within 24 hours.

☐ 5. All consultations not responded to within Emergency Center policy and procedure guidelines.

☐ 6. Misdiagnosis with adverse effects.

☐ 7. Patient leaves without being seen by a physician.

☐ 8. Patient/family complaint.

☐ 9. Other _____

Comments: _____

Helicopter/Ambulance Transports

☐ 10. Unnecessary delays with adverse effects.

☐ 11. Personnel problems resulting in delay of care or adverse patient outcome.

☐ 12. Patient family facility complaints.

☐ 13. Mechanical failure.

☐ 14. Scene time greater than 30 minutes.

☐ 15. Unresolved control problems at scene/accident resulting in delay of care.

☐ 16. Other _____

Comments: _____

Physician Response Required for Severity of Injury Marked Major, If Death Occurs or If Person Responsible for Completing Report Is Unable To Determine The Severity of Injury.

Name of
Physician Notified: _____ Time Notified: _____ Time Responded: _____

Physician Response: _____

Signature of Physician: _____   Ext./Beeper #

Brief Objective Description: (Should be factual information only. Include vital signs, follow-up care, x-rays, lab. etc.)_____

Person Completing Report (Signature):	Ext./Beeper#	Witness(es):	Ext./Beeper#
		a. _____	
		b. _____	
Manager/Supervisor (Signature):	Ext./Beeper#	Responsible Party or Department:	
Quality Assurance/Risk Management:	Date of Review:	PCE: ☐ YES ☐ NO	Comment(s): a. _____ b. _____

Figure 6.T. Incident report (also known as management variance report) used in an emergency department to collect data on a single sentinel event. Staff complete the form mainly by checking alternatives. This sample form is designed to allow a computer scanner to automatically enter its data into a computer system. Staff must be reassured that incident reports are needed to help mitigate or prevent future patient injuries, not to lay blame or to criticize.
Source: *University Hospital & Clinics, Columbia, Missouri. Used with permission.*

Report of Occurrences

1/6/89   MMA Computer Systems   QUALITY ASSURANCE

10:28 AM   **CONFIDENTIAL**

Report of Occurrences Attributed to Physicians by Medical Service
Reporting Period: May 1, 1988 through May 31, 1989

							MEDICAL SERVICE CODE: MED	INTERNAL MEDICINE				
PHYS. No.	PA-TIENT No.	OCCUR. DATE	CRITE-RION No.	ATTRI-BUTIONS	SEVERITY OF OCCUR.	STAN-DARD OF CARE	DESCRIPTION OF OCCURRENCE	AGE	FULL RECORD REVWD.	REPORT RISK MGMT.	REPORT COMM./ DEPT.
2114	1074377	5/5/88	2	2114 PHY	3	QUESTIN	Description of Occurrence: Readmit 12 hrs post-op w/fever & dyspnea. Adm note states "r/o pneumothorax s/p bronchoscopy." CXR confirmed pneumothorax. Chest tube inserted, pt stable.	55	Yes	Yes	Yes
							Physician Review: Readmit and care appropriate; however, pt should have been more thoroughly evaluated prior to discharge.				
							Quality Assurance Committee: Risk Mgt in contact w/family, & they are thankful for care pt received upon readmit. Chart breach of procedure during bronchoscopy. Noted that SDS dept busy/ short on staff. Recommend acuity studies be implemented re: better planning for staffing.				
4655	18992847	7/20/88	19B	4655 PHY	2	MET	Description of Occurrence: As of 11/20 LOS over avg & IS criteria not met. AP notified potential denial situation. No ECF beds available at this time.				
							Physician Review: IS criteria confirmed as not met. Agreed transfer to ECF appropriate. Family conference X3 led to transfer to ECF 12/2/87.				

FIGURE 6.U. *Form to record occurrence of sentinel events, including severity of occurrence, description of the occurrence, and other information.*
SOURCE: *Leahy MA, Tribbey MM: MMA computer systems. QRC Advisor 5(9):6, July 1989.*

Data Organization Table

Indicator	Number of Patients	Complying with Indicator	Percentage	Threshold for Evaluation	Threshold Reached
1	12	12	100%	95%	No
2	12	12	100%	95%	No
3	12	12	100%	95%	No
4	12	12	100%	95%	No
5	10	8	80%	90%	Yes (−10%)
6	12	7	58%	95%	Yes (−37%)
7	12	8	67%	95%	Yes (−28%)
8	10	7	70%	90%	Yes (−20%)

FIGURE 6.V. Table displays monitoring findings for eight indicators, showing in each case whether the threshold for evaluation was reached (ie, triggered). These results show that the thresholds for Indicators 1 through 4 were not reached, but those for Indicators 5 through 8 were.

An Example of Unit Monthly Report Data (Unit A)*

	Threshold for Evaluation	1 May	2 June	3 July	4 Aug	5 Sept	6 Oct
Psychiatric emergencies requiring temporary transfer of client to another facility	1	0	1	**5**	1	1	0
Behavior management incidents	3	3	**8**	**7**	**5**	3	2
Positions vacant at end of month							
Full-time vacancies	1	1	**3**	**2**	1	1	0
Part-time vacancies	1	1	**2**	**2**	1	1	0
Sick days used by staff	5	**8**	**9**	3	5	4	2
Clients' unauthorized absences	1	1	**5**	**3**	**3**	1	0
Abuse/neglect allegations reported	0	0	0	**1**	**1**	0	0
Client/student grievances	1	0	1	**3**	**2**	1	0

*Occurrences that exceed the threshold for evaluation are in **boldface**.*

FIGURE 6.W. Similar to Figure 6.V., this table tabulates data collected for several indicators and shows whether data collected during six monitoring periods reached (ie, triggered) thresholds for evaluation. *SOURCE: Vermillion JM, Pfeiffer SI: Unit-based clinical and organizational indicators for residential treatment. QRB 16(8):291, Aug 1990.*

Medical Record Completion Timeliness Monitors: Sample of _____ Records Reviewed Each Quarter

MONITOR	DESCRIPTION	THRESHOLD FOR EVALUATION	HOSPITAL PERFORMANCE			
			Jan-Mar	Apr-Jun	Jul-Sep	Oct-Dec
Average # of days record held in transcription area (awaiting dictation typing)	Total # of days record held in *transcription area* Total records reviewed					
Average # days between discharge and final filing of record	Total # days between discharge *and final filing of record* Total records reviewed					
% of history and physicals dictated prior to admission or within 24 hours of admission	# Hps dictated prior to or *within 24 hours of admission* Total records reviewed					
% of discharge summaries dictated within 15 days of discharge	# disch. summaries dictated *within 15 days of discharge* Total records reviewed					
Average # of unsigned orders at discharge	*Total # of unsigned orders* Total records reviewed					
Average # of DRG attestation statements signed within one week	Total number of DRG attestation *signed within one week* Total attestation statements run					

FIGURE 6.X. *Form to show monitored data levels (in this case, concerning medical records) by quarter year intervals.*
SOURCE: *Indicators of quality for medical record review.* QA Section Connection *(AMRA) 7(3):3, May/June 1989.*

Quality Monitoring Analysis Monthly Report

Persons in Attendance _____

_____

_____   Month_____

_____   Unit_____

Indicator	# Charts Reviewed	Compliance ① | ② | ③	Current Compliance Rate	% Change

Discussion:

Proposed actions:

Conclusion:

Indicator	# Charts Reviewed	Compliance ① | ② | ③	Current Compliance Rate	% Change

Discussion:

Proposed actions:

Conclusion:

Indicator	# Charts Reviewed	Compliance ① | ② | ③	Current Compliance Rate	% Change

Discussion:

Proposed actions:

Conclusion:

FIGURE 6.Y. *Brief report displays current compliance rate for specific indicators and percent of change since previous monitoring periods. This form could also be compactly presented in a column format.*

Perioperative Mortality

Hospital _____   Reporting Period (Quarter/Year): _____/_____

DATA ELEMENTS	TOTAL NUMBERS FOR THE QUARTER	RATE
1. Total number of procedures (OR and DR)	ASA Classification — 1, 2, 3, 4, 5, Total / Non-emergency / Emergency	
2. Total number of perioperative deaths within 48 hours of surgical procedure	ASA Classification — 1, 2, 3, 4, 5, Total / Non-emergency / Emergency	
3. Total perioperative mortality rate (total number of perioperative deaths divided by the total number of procedures, by category)		ASA Classification — 1, 2, 3, 4, 5, Total / Non-emergency / Emergency
4. Total number of perioperative deaths where anesthesia was administered by anesthesia staff		
5. Anesthesia perioperative mortality rate (total number of perioperative deaths where anesthesia was administered by anesthesia staff divided by the total number of procedures)		
6. Total number of perioperative deaths where anesthesia conducted a pre-operative assessment		
7. Preoperative assessment mortality rate (total number of perioperative deaths where anesthesia conducted a preop assessment divided by the total number of procedures)		

Comments:

FIGURE 6.Z. Form to display perioperative mortality. Several of the categories ask for data to be broken out by the anesthesiology (ASA) risk levels developed by the American Society of Anesthesiologists. SOURCE: Maryland Hospital Association Quality Indicator Project, 1991. Used with permission.

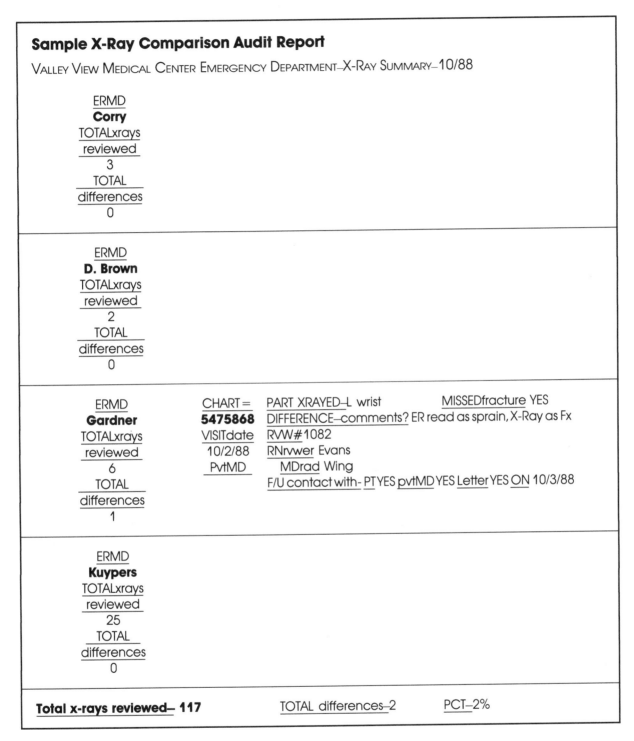

FIGURE 6.AA. *X-ray comparison audit report presents differences in scores between a physician's reading and a cardiologist's or radiologist's interpretation.*
SOURCE: *Keypers ME: A computerized log and integrated quality assessment program for the small emergency department. QRB 15(5):150, May 1989.*

Sample Blood Usage Report—Summary by Physician

PHYSICIAN ID: _____

Patient ID	Date Ordered	Component Ordered	Units Ordered	Units Given	Units Returned
_____	_____	_____	_____	_____	_____
_____	_____	_____	_____	_____	_____
_____	_____	_____	_____	_____	_____
_____	_____	_____	_____	_____	_____

Units Wasted	Own Blood	Indicator	Indicator Met	Reaction Code
_____	_____	_____	_____	_____
_____	_____	_____	_____	_____
_____	_____	_____	_____	_____
_____	_____	_____	_____	_____

FIGURE 6.BB. *Report form used to present summary information on blood use for an individual physician.*

Indexes of Patients' Ratings of Hospitalization

INDEX	DISTRIBUTION OF RESPONSES BY PERCENTAGE				
	HIGH				LOW
1. Satisfaction with preadmission information on medical care and costs	3	0	56	36	15
2. Satisfaction with preadmission information on hospital procedure	69	—	8	—	23
3. Satisfaction with hospital food	44	21	—	19	16
4. Satisfaction with physician	56	—	36	—	8
5. Discomfort/worry	24	18	27	20	12
6. Irritation	2	8	—	22	68
7. Satisfaction with information about illness while in hospital	63	17	9	7	5
8. Satisfaction with information about illness after discharge	75	13	—	5	6
9. Likelihood of future use of medical center	83	—	7	—	10

FIGURE 6.CC. *When data are composed of a range of more than two possible scores, data may be presented in a distribution table such as this.*
SOURCE: *Adapted from Houston CS, Pasanen WE: Patient perceptions of hospital care.* Hospitals *46(3):71-73, April 16, 1972.*

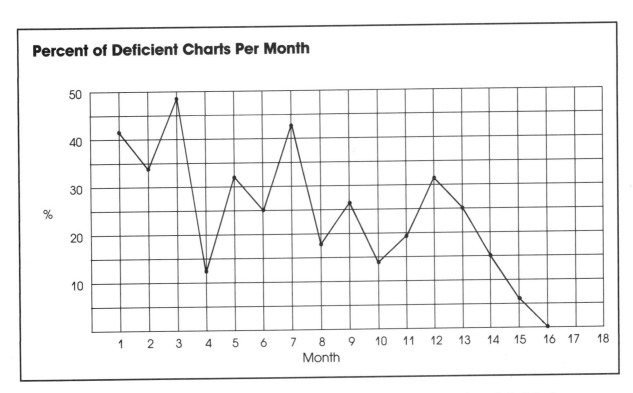

FIGURE 6.DD. *Data may also be organized graphically. (See Figures 7.W. through 7.OO. for many more examples of graphic presentation of data). Here the percentage of charts judged deficient varies from month to month depending upon the practitioner mix and the combination of indicators triggered in any given month.*
SOURCE: *Larsen RD, Bennion SD, Leonard TE: Monitoring and evaluation in an army health clinic. QRB 15(8):245, Aug 1989.*

Tabulation Worksheet—Patient Meal Surveys By Diet

Special Diets _____   Date: _____ Quarter: _____
or   Account Location: _____
Regular Diets _____   Profit Center: _____

Question #	(A) Excellent	(B) Very Good	(C) Good	(D) Fair	(E) Poor	(F) Total Responses	(G) Total Acceptable (A + B)	% A + B (G ÷ F × 100)
1.								
2.								
3.								
4.								
5.								
6.								
7.								
8.								
9.								*goal = 90% or better
10.								
11.								
12.								
13.								
14.								

Remarks: _____   Completed By: _____   Date: _____

FIGURE 6.EE. *Worksheet for tabulating results of a food service satisfaction survey. (The survey itself is shown as Figure 4.BB.)*
SOURCE: Marriott Quality Improvement Manual. *Washington, DC: Marriott Corp, 1990, p 72.*

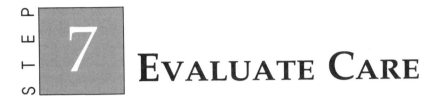

EVALUATE CARE

A decision must be made whether the data, both from ongoing monitoring and other quality-related feedback, warrant initiation of further evaluation of the aspect of care and service.

The findings from ongoing monitoring that show thresholds have been reached should be assessed, as well as other feedback (for example, patient satisfaction surveys, staff comments) that suggests opportunities for improvement may be present. Then, taking into consideration the potential effect on patient care and services as well as organization resources, priorities for further evaluation are set.

When collected data reach the threshold for evaluation, staff members with expertise in the particular areas assessed must evaluate the care provided to determine whether actions to improve care should be taken. This evaluation usually includes searching for patterns or trends in patient care that cause delays, undesired variations in outcome, lack of continuity of care, or other problems. Patterns such as periodic inadequate staffing levels may relate to specific units, personnel, clinical functions, segments of the patient population, or other factors. Determining the patterns of care that caused the threshold for evaluation to be reached may often be more valuable in improving overall care than will the findings of peer reviewers looking at individual cases.

No change in order to improve should be made until (1) the current processes are understood, and (2) evaluation indicates how the current processes can be improved. Even when the quality of care and services meet current expectations, opportunities to improve care may be identified.

THE TEAM APPROACH

Those individuals who can best evaluate all facets of the particular aspect(s) of care and service may be brought together. This "team" may be the team who developed the indicators and thresholds, or another group with appropriate representation. When necessary, these teams should be composed of members from different departments and services, to assure that interdepartmental processes are considered.

TOOLS FOR EVALUATING CARE

The actual process of evaluating care involves breaking out the data in practitioners, various ways to see which processes, departments, shifts, practitioners, or other factors have contributed most to the rate of indicator occurrences and exactly what, when, and where the opportunity for improvement is.

One difficulty in evaluating care and service is determining exactly how performance can be improved. It is important to make such decisions as objectively as possible. Many tools can help assure objectively and to understand the causes of observed performance; these include

Eight Helpful Charts

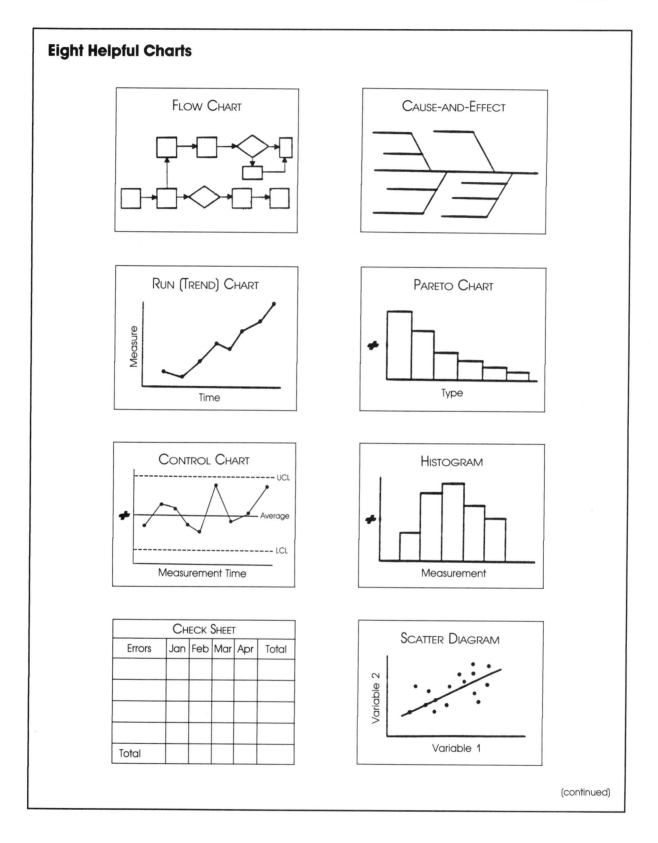

(continued)

Eight Helpful Charts (continued)

Technique Selection Guide

Task	Techniques
1. To decide which problem will be addressed first (or next)	• Flow Chart • Check Sheet • Pareto Chart
2. To arrive at a statement that describes the problem in terms of what it is specifically, where it occurs, when it happens, and its extent	• Check Sheet • Pareto Chart • Run Chart • Histogram • Pie Chart
3. To develop a complete picture of all the possible causes of the problem	• Check Sheet • Cause & Effect Diagram
4. To agree on the basic cause(s) of the problem	• Check Sheet • Pareto Chart • Scatter Diagram
5. To implement the solution and establish needed monitoring procedures and charts	• Pareto Chart • Histogram • Control Chart

Source: Brassard M: The Memory Jogger: A Pocket Guide of Tools for Continuous Improvement, *2nd ed, Methuen, MA: Goal/QPC, 1988, p 31.*

measures of processes and outcomes; cause-and-effect diagrams, Pareto diagrams, flow charts, run charts, control charts, histograms, and scatter diagrams; department standards, guidelines, protocols, and parameters of care or practice; the team members' expertise; professional society guidelines and standards; and pertinent health care literature.

Graphs or narrative summaries may be of use to display or explain findings, as well as to report historical trends. Graphic displays can often get the attention of administrative and clinical decision makers much better than pages of discussion. Graphic representations of QA data—objective and succinct—are often especially appealing to physicians.

When it is appropriate to conduct an intensive review of occurrences related to a particular practitioner, peer review is undertaken. In such cases, peer review is a critical element in the monitoring and evaluation process; the productivity of this intensive use of professionals' time can be increased through the use of indicator data and associated thresholds for evaluation to identify cases for review.

An important shift in emphasis

In the past, monitoring and evaluation has often focused on finding the "bad apples"—practitioners not performing up to standards. Certainly, one component of improving quality must be to help find and solve the chronic problems, whether those problems are systems, equipment, or personnel. But the greatest opportunities to improve the quality of care and service do not lie in the errors people make—rather, they lie in improving the overall performance of the systems, equipment, and personnel—the continuous improvement of performance; opportunities for such improvement are most often found in ongoing processes rather than in isolated individuals.

The following section, comprising tables, forms, graphs, and charts used in trend analysis, is perhaps the most important in this publication. Trend analysis is the process of organizing indicator occurrence data by practitioner, shift, facility, or other variable to shed light on patterns of care and identify aspects of care needing improvement. The process focuses on isolating reasons why indicator occurrence rates exceeded their thresholds for evaluation. In the process, underlying causes for variation in patient care are highlighted, and actions designed to improve care are planned.

Figures 7.A. through 7.W. show ways to organize data to highlight underlying care patterns. Data can be arranged by type of indicator occurrence, department in which occurrences were noted, severity of illness, staff member responsible, day of the week, unit or room, shift, hospital (when data is available to compare one hospital to others), and so on. Computing of standard deviations may also be helpful in showing where a given finding falls within a spectrum of variance (see Figures 7.B., 7.C., B.5., and especially Appendix C, page 279). At the heart of this section, five case histories (Figures 7.S. through 7.W.) show how evaluation can look at a single situation in many ways in order to find underlying opportunities for improvement. Figures 7.V. and 7.W. show how graphic tools can be used to bring out otherwise "hidden" patterns of care.

New ways to display data graphically in order to highlight trends or report findings to staff and management continue to emerge and evolve. In general, charts and other graphic devices are effective ways to complement narrative or numerical reporting, enhancing their power of explanation and persuasion. The nine uses of graphics, according to one source, are to

1. enhance clarity,

2. simplify,

3. give emphasis,

4. summarize,

5. reinforce,

6. enhance interest,

7. increase impact,

8. increase credibility, and

9. help put many facts into an understandable, coordinated whole that hangs together.[1]

Included as Figures 7.X. through 7.GG. are several graphic possibilities (also see Figures 7.N., 7.U., and 7.V.). These include bar, line, and pie charts.

Also included are examples of the eight graphic tools most often associated with a continuous quality improvement approach to addressing quality of care (see the Introduction for a brief discussion of continous quality improvement). These tools are

- process flow charts (Figure 7.HH.),

- run charts (Figure 7.II.),

- control charts (Figure 7.JJ.),

- cause-and-effect diagrams (Figure 7.KK.),

- Pareto charts (Figure 7.LL.),

- histograms (Figure 7.MM.),

- check sheets (Figure 7.NN.), and
- scatter diagrams (Figure 7.OO.).

A brief description of each tool is included. (How to create and use control charts, in particular, is discussed in some detail in Appendix C, page 279.)

These are tools used to understand patient care processes and to help ensure objectivity in assessing the causes of observed patterns of performance. (See the accompanying figure for a schematic representation of these tools and a table of tasks each is used to accomplish.)

The level of mathematics necessary to use these tools "is no more than a seventh or eight grader might learn," writes Mary Walton. "Several of the basic tools are merely ways of organizing and visually displaying data. In most cases, employees can collect the data and do much of the interpretation."[2]

Basing improvements on data and statistical analysis is central to a continuous quality improvement approach. "Statistical methods help to understand processes, to bring them under control, and then to improve them," continues Walton. "Otherwise, people will forever be 'putting out fires' rather than improving the system."[2] Basing decisions on objective data also helps avoid basing them on mere hunches and mistaken impressions.

Finally, Figures 7.PP. through 7.VV. are forms and tables designed to help document or think through the evaluation process. These include forms to evaluate individual cases through peer review.

References

1. Lefferts R: *How to Prepare Charts and Graphs for Effective Reports.* New York: Barnes & Noble Books, 1982, p 19.

2. Walton M: *The Deming Management Method.* New York: Dodd, Mead & Co, Inc, 1986, pp 96-97.

Algorithm Tracking Tool (Patient Incident Statistics)

Unit _____

Month Shift	Quarter _____			_____			_____			_____		
	1st	2nd	3rd	1st	2nd	3rd	1st	2nd	3rd	1st	2nd	3rd
TOTAL-All Incidents												
MEDICATION ERRORS — Number												
Patient — Lack of Knowledge												
Patient — Disregard for Rules												
Patient — Need for Control												
Nurse — Lack of Knowledge												
Nurse — Assessment/Intervention												
Nurse — Noncompliance												
Other Dept.												
Significance*												
Equip. — Not Available												
Equip. — Failure to Function												
PATIENT FALLS — Number												
Patient — Lack of Knowledge												
Patient — Disregard for Rules												
Patient — Need for Control												
Nurse — Lack of Knowledge												
Nurse — Assessment/Intervention												
Nurse — Noncompliance												
Other Dept.												
Significance*												
Equip. — Not Available												
Equip. — Failure to Function												
OTHER INCIDENTS — Number												
Patient — Lack of Knowledge												
Patient — Disregard for Rules												
Patient — Need for Control												
Nurse — Lack of Knowledge												
Nurse — Assessment/Intervention												
Nurse — Noncompliance												
Other Dept.												
Significance*												
Equip. — Not Available												
Equip. — Failure to Function												

*Significance: Identify those incidents that caused potential or actual injury to patient.

FIGURE 7.A. A form to trend patient incidents by type of incident, reason for the incident, shift, and month.
SOURCE: St Mary's Hospital, Milwaukee. Used with permission.

Table Showing Distribution of All Hospitals For the Quarter

	Indicators	− Outliers	− 2SD	− 1SD	Mean	+ 1SD	+ 2SD	+ Outliers
I	Hosp Acq Infec		A B F K	C L P N	7.5%	E G J M	H I	O
II	Surg Wound Infec		N O	D F G H I K L M	26.7%	A C J	B P	E
III	Inpat Mortality		B H J K	F I N	13.2%	G L O	A M P	C D E
IV	Neo Mortality		B	A	21.5%	C	M	P
V	Perio Mortality			B H I K M	12.0%	A G J N P	C F L	D E O
VI	Cesarean Sec			B E F G K O P	15.4%	A H J L N	C I M	D
VII	Unplanned Readmi		C K M	F L	10.9%	G H I	J	A
VIII	Unp Adm Fol Ambu			B C D E J L O	8.7%	A G I K P	F M N	H
IX	Unp Ret To SCU	A H	C G	D E I P	4.8%	B J K L N	F M	O
X	Unp Ret To OR			A C D E F J M P	9.2%	G H I K N O	B L	
Letters refer to hospitals								

Figure 7.B. *When comparing several hospitals, practitioners, or departments, each one may be ranked by where it falls within a standard deviation spectrum. In general, standard deviation analysis is a useful tool for identifying outliers. A numerical percentage shows the mean for each indicator; the identification code letter of each participating hospital is included in the appropriate boxes according to how their indicator rates compare to the mean. Values and hospital codes shown have been created for purposes of this example.*
Source: *Maryland Hospital Association Quality Indicator Project, 1991. Used with permission.*

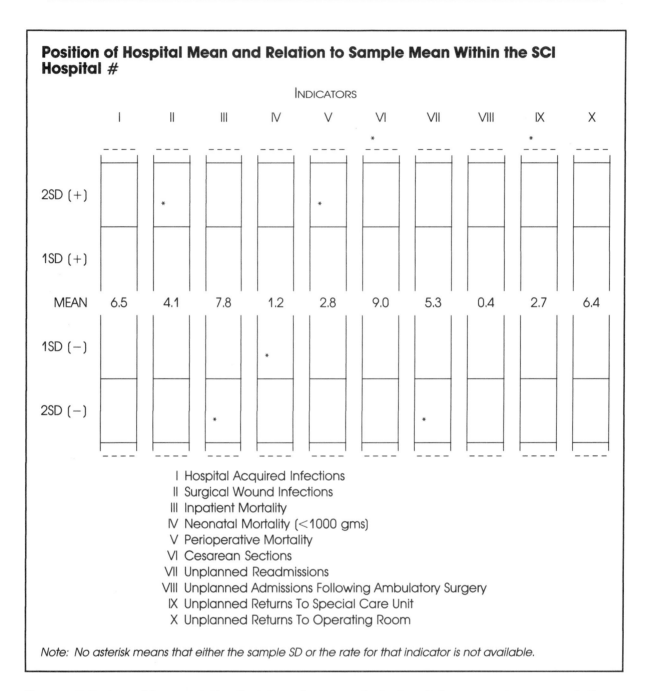

FIGURE 7.C. A graphic presentation that shows how a particular hospital compares to a group of other hospitals in its rate of indicator compliance. The asterisk represents the hospital's indicator rate. Values shown have been created for purposes of this example.
SOURCE: Maryland Hospital Association Quality Indicator Project, 1991. Used with permission.

Quality Indicator Report

Obstetrics
Hospital: No Name Available
Region: North Central
Current Time Period: 07/90 – 09/90
Previous Time Period: 04/90 – 06/90

Indicator	Hospital					Region			Total U.S.		
	Current		Previous		Signif	Number	%	Signif	Number	%	Signif
	Number	%	Number	%							
Total obstetric patients	1,607		1,539			1,602,160			4,875,835		
Abortion patients	14	.9	13	.8		52,139	3.3		135,624	2.8	
OB, Not delivered	129	8.0	127	8.3		181,910	11.4		591,747	12.1	
OB, Delivered	1,443	89.8	1,371	89.1		1,330,794	83.1		4,039,568	82.8	
Vaginal delivery patients	1,158	80.2	1,088	79.4		964,504	72.5		3,058,027	75.7	
C-Section delivery patients	285	19.8	283	20.6		366,289	27.5		981,541	24.3	
1. Obstetric patients, expired	2	.1			?	311		?	809		?
2. OB PT misadventures			1	.1		2,204	.1		5,385	.1	
Age < 18 years, with CC code						36			118		
Age < 18 years, with no CC code									13		
Age 18–40 years, with CC code						1,745	.1		4,235	.1	
Age 18–40 years, with no CC code			1	.1		369			939		
Age > 40 years, with CC code						53			78		
Age > 40 years, with no CC code											
3. Number of ectopic pregnancies	18	1.1	23	1.5		26,395	1.6		78,683	1.6	
4. Number of incomplete abortions	8	57.1	9	69.2		35,724	68.5		92,722	68.4	
5. Legally induced abortions	2	14.3			>	9,086	17.4		19,379	14.3	
6. Legally induced abortion w/infection						420	4.6		1,047	5.4	
7. Legally induced abortion w/hemorrhage						476	5.2		1,054	5.4	
8. Failed abortion attempts						183	.4		476	.4	
9. OB PTS with postpartum complications	138	9.5	130	9.4		78,104	5.8	?	323,160	7.9	?
Age < 18 years, with CC code			1	.1		3,571	.3	+	10,848	.3	+
Age < 18 years, with no CC code	1	.1	2	.1		2,859	.2		7,108	.2	
Age 18–40 years, with CC code	45	3.1	43	3.1		36,474	2.7		163,337	4.0	+
Age 18–40 years, with no CC code	91	6.3		6.0		34,481	2.6	?	138,990	3.4	?
Age > 40 years, with CC code	1	.1			?	382			1,527		
Age > 40 years, with no CC code			1	.1		335			1,348		

The "?", "+", ">", and "<" indicate a statistically significant (P < 0.05) difference from the relevant norm.

"Blank" indicates no significant difference from the relevant norm.

? indicates a difference suggestive of a lower level of quality (ie, more hospital incurred trauma).

+ indicates the difference is suggestive of higher quality (ie, fewer medical misadventures).

> indicates a statistically significant difference, greater than the relevant norm, with no clear implication for hospital quality (ie, more patients with a length of stay of one day or less).

< indicates a statistically significant difference, lower than the relevant norm, with no clear implication for hospital quality (ie, fewer patients admitted from a skilled nursing facility).

Figure 7.D. Table helps compare a hospital's current indicator rate to its previous rate, the rate of other hospital's in the region, and total U.S. rate. The "significance" columns use symbols to show whether there is a difference in any two rates suggestive of a lower or higher level of quality at the hospital. Values shown have been created for purposes of this example.
Source: Healthcare Knowledge Resources, Ann Arbor, MI, 1991. Used with permission.

Perinatal Morbidity and Mortality

Data are for 19 _____
Quarter _____

	Birth weights (g)							
	501-749	750-999	1,000-1,249	1,250-1,499	1,500-1,999	2,000-2,499	>2,500	Total for all weights
Number of births (all)								
Number of perinatal deaths (fetal and neonatal deaths)								
Fetal deaths Antepartum								
Intrapartum								
Neonatal deaths (<28 days)								
Total perinatal mortality rate = Number of perinatal deaths / Number of all births								_____%
Neonatal autopsies performed								
Birth trauma (all types)								

Figure 7.E. *Form illustrates how occurrences of perinatal mortality can be grouped by neonate birthweight.*
Source: *American College of Obstetricians and Gynecologists (ACOG) Task Force:* Quality Assurance in Obstetrics and Gynecology. *Washington, DC: ACOG, 1989, p 95.*

Correlations with Overall Satisfaction

	Medical Patients	Surgical Patients	Obstetric Patients
Satisfaction scale			
Doctor satisfaction	.72*	.41*	.46*
Nursing satisfaction	.76*	.52*	.51*
Labor and delivery nursing satisfaction	n/a	n/a	.41*
Room satisfaction	.41*	.56*	.50*
Food satisfaction	.49*	.47*	.43*
Pain control	n/a	.44*	n/a
Thought length of stay was too long	.06	−.03	.04
Patient characteristics			
Income	.02	.00	.00
Perceived health	.36*	.25*	.18*
Emergency admission	.02	.03	n/a
Length of stay	.01	−.05	.09
*p<.01			

FIGURE 7.F. *Tables can also trend data by type of patient. Table shows the correlation coefficient of satisfaction survey results and type of patient.*
SOURCE: *Cleary PD, et al: Patient assessments of hospital care. QRB 15(6):178, June 1989.*

Daily ED Time Study: Length of Treatment

TREATMENT TIMES:	LESS THAN 2 HR			2-4 HR			OVER 4 HR			LEFT WITHOUT BEING SEEN		
Shifts:	7-3	3-11	11-7	7-3	3-11	11-7	7-3	3-11	11-7	7-3	3-11	11-7
No. of patients												
Percent patients by shift												
Percent patients by category												
Total percent												

FIGURE 7.G. *Length of treatment is broken out by shift in this form.*
SOURCE: *Allegheny General Hospital, Pittsburgh. Used with permission.*

Distribution of Errors by Disease Category (N = 146)

NUMBER (PERCENT) OF CASES PER DISEASE CATEGORY

PATIENT MANAGEMENT ERROR	RECURRENT HEART FAILURE	RECURRENT TRANSIENT ISCHEMIC ATTACK	RECURRENT CEREBROVASCULAR ACCIDENT	GASTROINTESTINAL HEMMORRHAGE	ACUTE BACTERIAL PNEUMONIA
Insufficient date acquisition	10 (22)	6 (27)	3 (15)	2 (18)	1 (10)
Inadequate hypothesis generation	23 (51)	6 (32)	6 (30)	3 (27)	1 (10)
Inattention or misinterpretation of cues	14 (31)	7 (32)	10 (50)	2 (18)	2 (20)
Inattention to or mismanagement of therapy	15 (33)	3 (14)	4 (20)	1 (9)	4 (40)
Delayed or missed diagnosis	8 (18)	1 (5)	0 (0)	0 (0)	0 (0)
Delayed treatment	9 (20)	2 (10)	2 (10)	1 (9)	1 (10)

FIGURE 7.H. *Indicator occurrence data trended by disease category.*
SOURCE: *Weinberg NS: The relation of medical problem solving and therapeutic errors to disease categories. QRB 15(9):269, Sept 1989.*

Occurrence Summary Report

1/4/89   MMA Computer Systems   QUALITY ASSURANCE

12:36 p.m.   **CONFIDENTIAL**

Occurrence Summary Report—Medical Service

Reporting Period: April 1, 1987 Through March 31, 1989

Key
PO = Patient Occurrence
RDD = Record Documentation Deficiency
UR = Utilization Review

MEDICAL SERVICE CODE: MED   DESCRIPTION: INTERNAL MEDICINE

Indicator Number	Indicator Type	Total	_ Severity of Occurrence _											_ Standard of Care _				
			1	2	3	4	5	0	RDD			Other	MET	NOTMET	QUESTN		Other
1	PO	52	31	16	2	1	2						37	4	11		
2	PO	84	47	23	10		1	3					62	13	9		
3	RDD	872							872								872
4	PO	76	30	32	4	7	1	1				1	53	7	16		
5	PO	8		3	4							1	1	4	3		
6	PO	15	13	2									13	1	1		
7	PO	23	11	7	3	1	1						11	6	6		
8	PO	76	59	12		2		3					49	7	20		
9	PO	176	49	63	31	23	10						87	31	58		
10	PO	80	15	23	12	18	12						62	6	12		
11	PO	28	17	11									17	6	5		
12	PO	92	37	15	19	8	6	7					74	5	13		
13	PO	36	21	7	6	2							20	2	14		
14	PO	84	32	27	18		6					1	57	13	14		
15	PO	52	47	1	4								47	2	3		
16	PO	7	1	4	1	1							3	2	2		
17	PO	208					208						174	7	27		
18	PO	41	27	14									34	5	2		
19	UR	104	18	27	3			56					97	2	5		
20	RDD	406							406								406
21	RDD	374							374								374
22	PO	9	1					8					6	1	2		
23	PO	15						13				2	13		2		
24	UR	66										66					66
Page Totals:		2984	456	287	117	63	250	88	1652	0	0	71	917	124	225	0	1718
Medical Service Total:		2984	456	287	117	63	250	88	1652	0	0	71	917	124	225	0	1718
Percent:			15.3	9.6	3.9	2.1	8.4	3.0	55.4	0.0	0.0	2.3	30.7	4.2	7.5	0.0	57.6

FIGURE 7.I. Indicator occurrences grouped by severity of illness level. In order to make this table more intelligible for staff members and administrators, the indicator codes (first two vertical columns) might be replaced by written-out indicators.
SOURCE: Adapted from Leahy MA, Tribbey MM: MMA computer systems. QRC Advisor 5(9):5, July 1989.

Importance of Severity of Illness in Explaining Variations in Charges for Selected Heterogeneous DRGs

	Variation in Charges (SD)	Percentage of Variation in Charges Explained			Contribution of Severity to Explanation‡
		Discrete Explanations*		Interactive Explanation†	
		LOS	Severity	LOS and Severity	
DRG 374—adverse effect of drug, toxic effect of alcohol, without secondary diagnosis					
(N = 16)	$1,548	30.2‖	43.5‖	59.7‖	28.8§
Severity class					
I (n = 1)	—		2.3		<0.1
II (n = 13)	596		22.6§		35.4‖
IV (n = 2)	4,984		44.9‖		49.8‖
DRG 202—abdominal hernia except simple inguinal of ages 14-64, with major repair					
(N = 27)	$2,176	86.7‖	64.9‖	87.7‖	7.7
Severity class					
I (n = 5)	664		5.4		1.4
II (n = 19)	1,917		11.2		6.3
III (n = 1)	—		<0.1		2.4
IV (n = 2)	6,398		89.1‖		55.4‖
DRG 132—heart failure without operation					
(N = 64)	$1,323	74.9‖	13.4‖	77.7‖	11.4‖
Severity class					
II (n = 17)	885		7.0		3.5
III (n = 33)	1,191		0.2		1.6
IV (n = 13)	1,979		8.0		13.7‖

*Percentage of variance in charges explained by LOS or severity, respectively (squared zero order correlation coefficients, converted to percentages).

†Percentage of variance in charges explained by LOS and severity together (squared multiple correlation coefficient, converted to a percentage).

‡Percentage of unexplained variance in charges that is reduced by the addition of the severity variable (squared partial correlation coefficient, converted to a percentage).

§Significant at .05 level.

‖Significant at .01 level.

FIGURE 7.J. *The effect of severity of illness on variation in patient charges can be explored using the statistical technique of correlation coefficients.*
SOURCE: *Kreitzer SL, Loebner ES, Roveti GC: Severity of illness: The DRGs' missing link? QRB Special Edition, Spring 1983, p 83.*

Sample Indicator Monitoring Report—Departmental

Department: _____

Indicator Code: _____   Description: _____

Threshold: _____

Date of Report: _____/_____/_____   By: _____

	Department Total	Physician 1 (or Nurse, etc)	Physician 2 (or Nurse, etc)	Physician 3 (or Nurse, etc)	Physician 4 (or Nurse, etc)
Total Events Recorded	_____	_____	_____	_____	_____
Number Noncompliance	_____	_____	_____	_____	_____
Percent Noncompliance	_____	_____	_____	_____	_____
Threshold Reached (Y/N)	_____	_____	_____	_____	_____
Number Noncompliance Justified	_____	_____	_____	_____	_____

FIGURE 7.K. *Form trends indicator compliance by practitioner. To preserve confidentiality, individual QA codes can be substituted for each practitioner's name.*

Sample Physician Communication Profile

Below is a set of questions describing health care experiences. The patients were asked to respond to these questions based on their perceptions of Dr A's care using a scale from 5 (strongly agree) to 1 (strongly disagree). They were also given the option of choosing "not applicable."

Asterisks note significant differences between group mean and individual mean scores.
    $p < .05$*
    $p < .01$**

	MEAN SCORE DR A	GROUP MEAN	RANGE DR A
This physician . . .			
1. spends enough time with me.	4.12*	4.40	5.0-2.0
2. explains my condition or diagnosis to my satisfaction.	4.20	4.44	5.0-2.0
3. provides me with the results of lab tests or X-rays.	4.37	4.46	5.0-3.0
4. answers my questions.	4.37	4.46	5.0-3.0

5. Generally, how would you describe the quality of care you receive from Dr A?

Comments:

"Excellent. Dr A takes the time to answer all questions asked and never seems to be in a rush to go to another appointment."

"Very good. He is clear about diagnosis and options available. He gave me straightforward answers."

"He was very thorough when I was in the office but was less helpful over the phone."

"Difficult to assess. I feel my symptoms were treated, but my problem was not treated."

FIGURE 7.L. Form shows patients' mean satisfaction score related to a particular physician, compares it with the mean of the physician group, and shows the range of scores for the physician.
SOURCE: Kind EA: Quality assurance in the ambulatory setting. In Spath PL (ed): Innovations in Health Care Quality Measurement. *Chicago: American Hospital Publishing, 1989, p 123.*

Sample Two-Part Form for Trending Adverse Patient Occurrences by Individual Physician

PART I

Practitioner Code: _____   Reporting Period: _____

Indicator Number	Disch. Date	Coded Patient Identifier	Age	Sex	Brief Description of Occurrence	Severity Code	Guideline of Care			MD/Spec Record Review	Reported to QA Comm.	Reported to RM	Follow-up action	
							+	+/−	−				Y	N

PART II. CONFIDENTIAL QUALITY ASSURANCE REPORT FOR PEER REVIEW

Summary of Individual Physician APO Trend Analyses

Reporting Period: _____ to: _____

Phys. Code	# Pts. Disch. This Period	# Pts. with APOs	% Pts. with APOs	Total # APOs	APOs by Severity							APOs Reviewed for Guideline of Care			Action/Comments
					0	1	2	3	4	5	6	+	+/−	−	

FIGURE 7.M. *Two-part form for trending adverse patient occurrences by physician.*
SOURCE: *Adapted from Medical Management Analysis International, Inc, Auburn, CA, 1989. Used with permission.*

Frequency Table Comparing AMI Length of Stay for Physicians in Two Departments*

	DEPARTMENT OF MEDICINE			DEPARTMENT OF FAMILY PRACTICE		
AVERAGE LENGTH OF STAY (DAYS)	NUMBER OF PHYSICIANS	FREQUENCY	FREQUENCY %	NUMBER OF PHYSICIANS	FREQUENCY	FREQUENCY %
3	ЖĦ	5	19.2	I	1	5.9
4	I	1	3.8	II	2	11.8
5	ЖĦ IIII	9	34.6	ЖĦ II	7	41.2
6	II	2	7.7	ЖĦ I	6	35.2
7	I	1	3.8	I	1	5.9
8	II	2	7.7			
9	II	2	7.7			
10	I	1	3.8			
11	I	1	3.8			
12	I	1	3.8			
13						
14						
15	I	1	3.8			
Total	**26**	**26**	**100.0***	**17**	**17**	**100.0***

*Rounded.

Histogram Example Showing Average Length of Stay by Physician Provider in Two Departments

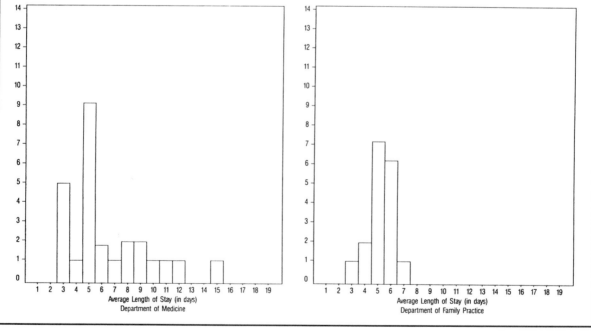

FIGURE 7.N. Frequency table and histogram showing length-of-stay patterns for physicians in two departments.
SOURCE: Longo DR, Ciccone KR, Lord JT: Integrated Quality Assessment: A Model for Concurrent Review, *Chicago: American Hospital Publishing, Inc, 1989, pp 136-137.*

Quality Assurance Report
Medical Records Department
Physician Specific Exception Distribution

Doctor	"N"	TIMELINESS OF COMPLETION								CLINICAL PERTINENCE					
		H & P		Prog Notes		Written Consult		OP Notes		Substantiation of Diagnosis		Abnormal Results		Content of Discharge Summary	
		#	%	#	%	#	%	#	%	#	%	#	%	#	%
1001	22	7	31.8	0	0.0	0	0.0	0	0.0	0	0.0	0	0.0	3	14.3
1003	6	1	16.7	0	0.0	0	0.0	0	0.0	0	0.0	0	0.0	0	0.0
1004	13	0	0.0	0	0.0	0	0.0	0	0.0	0	0.0	1	7.7	0	0.0
1011	13	4	30.8	0	0.0	0	0.0	0	0.0	0	0.0	0	0.0	0	0.0
1019	6	2	33.3	0	0.0	0	0.0	0	0.0	0	0.0	0	0.0	0	0.0
1025	13	1	7.7	0	0.0	0	0.0	0	0.0	0	0.0	1	7.7	0	0.0
1035	1	1	100	0	0.0	0	0.0	0	0.0	0	0.0	0	0.0	0	0.0
2026	16	1	6.3	0	0.0	0	0.0	0	0.0	0	0.0	0	0.0	0	0.0
2058	15	4	26.7	0	0.0	0	0.0	0	0.0	0	0.0	0	0.0	0	0.0
4003	13	2	15.4	1	7.7	0	0.0	0	0.0	0	0.0	0	0.0	0	0.0
4014	2	0	0.0	0	0.0	1	100	0	0.0	0	0.0	0	0.0	0	0.0
5008	10	0	0.0	0	0.0	3	50.0	1	25.0	0	0.0	0	0.0	0	0.0
5009	1	0	0.0	0	0.0	1	100	0	0.0	0	0.0	0	0.0	0	0.0
5021	8	0	0.0	0	0.0	0	0.0	1	25.0	0	0.0	0	0.0	0	0.0
7002	6	0	0.0	0	0.0	1	25.0	0	0.0	0	0.0	0	0.0	0	0.0
7007	2	1	50.0	0	0.0	0	0.0	0	0.0	0	0.0	0	0.0	2	100
8001	1	0	0.0	0	0.0	0	0.0	0	0.0	0	0.0	0	0.0	1	100
Department Rate		24	16.2	1	0.6	6	4.0	2	1.3	0	0.0	2	1.3	6	4.0

FIGURE 7.O. Table to show number and percentage of indicator occurrences for individual physicians. The table shows areas in which practitioners exhibit delinquencies in medical records.
SOURCE: Adapted from Quality Assurance Data Management in a Quality Improvement Environment *(Joint Commission binder book distributed at its 1990 educational conference "Quality Assurance Data Management—the Next Generation")*. Chicago: Joint Commission, 1990, chapter 5, p 26.

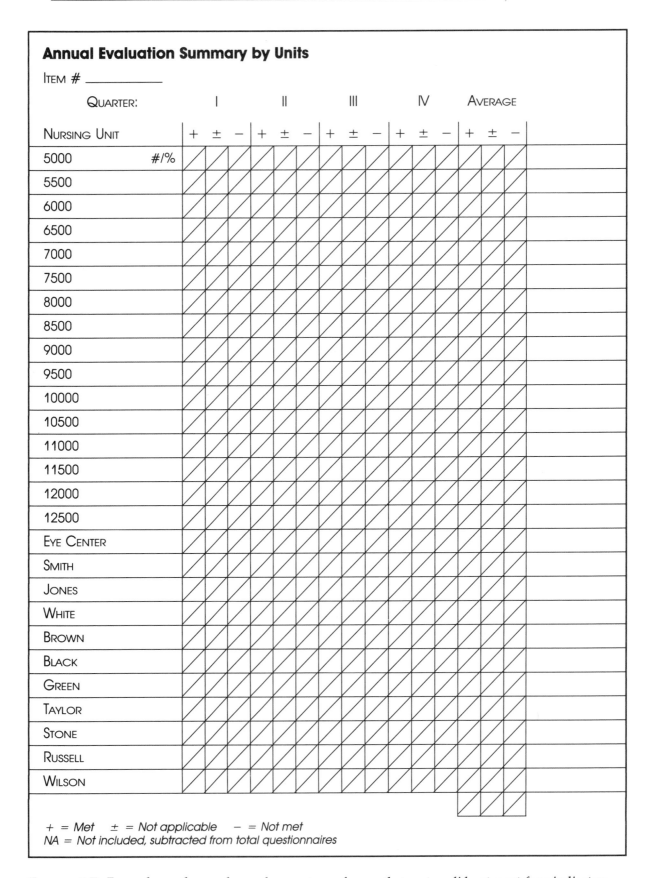

Annual Evaluation Summary by Units

Item # _____

Quarter:	I			II			III			IV			Average			
Nursing Unit	+	±	−	+	±	−	+	±	−	+	±	−	+	±	−	
5000 #/%																
5500																
6000																
6500																
7000																
7500																
8000																
8500																
9000																
9500																
10000																
10500																
11000																
11500																
12000																
12500																
Eye Center																
Smith																
Jones																
White																
Brown																
Black																
Green																
Taylor																
Stone																
Russell																
Wilson																

+ = Met   ± = Not applicable   − = Not met
NA = Not included, subtracted from total questionnaires

Figure 7.P. Form shows the number and percentage of cases that met or did not meet four indicators (trended by nursing unit and physician).

Profile of Critical Incident Reports

		Oct	Nov	Dec	Jan	Feb	Mar	Apr	May	Total
NUMBER OF CRITICAL INCIDENT REPORTS		4	7	4	8	12	14	19	17	85
PLACE OF INCIDENT	Unit A	1	1	0	1	3	3	4	2	15
	B	0	1	0	2	2	1	3	4	13
	C	2	0	1	1	1	2	3	2	12
	D	0	1	2	2	2	3	4	3	17
	Off unit	1	3	0	1	2	4	5	4	20
	Off grounds	0	1	1	1	2	1	0	2	8
NURSING SHIFT	Days	3	2	2	4	4	6	5	7	33
	Evenings	1	3	0	1	5	5	7	7	29
	Nights	0	2	2	3	3	3	7	3	23
NUMBER OF CRITICAL INCIDENTS BY PHYSICIAN	MD 1	1	0	1	0	1	0	2	1	6
	MD 2	0	1	1	2	1	2	1	0	8
	MD 3	1	2	1	1	2	3	5	1	16
	MD 4	0	0	0	1	1	2	1	2	7
	MD 5	0	1	0	0	1	0	2	2	6
	MD 6	1	0	0	0	1	0	1	3	6
	MD 7	0	1	0	1	2	3	3	1	11
	MD 8	1	0	1	1	2	0	2	3	10
	MD 9	0	0	0	0	1	2	2	4	9

FIGURE 7.Q. *A single matrix can trend for four or even more factors. This example provides an analysis of critical incidents by monthly number of incident reports, location of incidents, nursing shift, and physician.*

Quality-of-Care Measurement Laboratory Feedback Study
Executive Summary July 1991

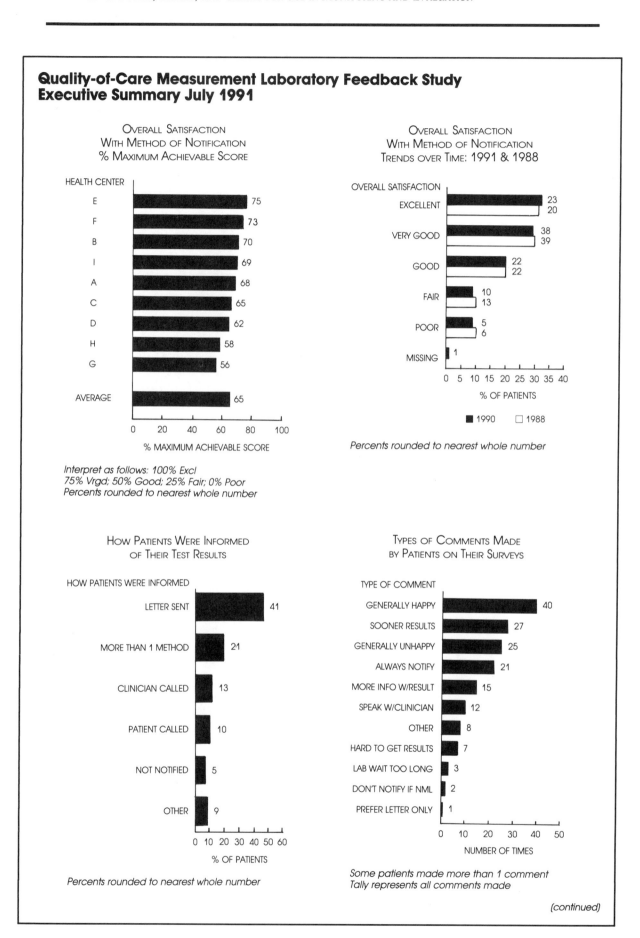

OVERALL SATISFACTION
WITH METHOD OF NOTIFICATION
% MAXIMUM ACHIEVABLE SCORE

HEALTH CENTER

E   75
F   73
B   70
I   69
A   68
C   65
D   62
H   58
G   56

AVERAGE   65

0   20   40   60   80   100
% MAXIMUM ACHIEVABLE SCORE

Interpret as follows: 100% Excl
75% Vrgd; 50% Good; 25% Fair; 0% Poor
Percents rounded to nearest whole number

OVERALL SATISFACTION
WITH METHOD OF NOTIFICATION
TRENDS OVER TIME: 1991 & 1988

OVERALL SATISFACTION

EXCELLENT   23 / 20
VERY GOOD   38 / 39
GOOD   22 / 22
FAIR   10 / 13
POOR   5 / 6
MISSING   1

0   5   10   15   20   25   30   35   40
% OF PATIENTS

■ 1990   □ 1988

Percents rounded to nearest whole number

HOW PATIENTS WERE INFORMED
OF THEIR TEST RESULTS

HOW PATIENTS WERE INFORMED

LETTER SENT   41
MORE THAN 1 METHOD   21
CLINICIAN CALLED   13
PATIENT CALLED   10
NOT NOTIFIED   5
OTHER   9

0   10   20   30   40   50   60
% OF PATIENTS

Percents rounded to nearest whole number

TYPES OF COMMENTS MADE
BY PATIENTS ON THEIR SURVEYS

TYPE OF COMMENT

GENERALLY HAPPY   40
SOONER RESULTS   27
GENERALLY UNHAPPY   25
ALWAYS NOTIFY   21
MORE INFO W/RESULT   15
SPEAK W/CLINICIAN   12
OTHER   8
HARD TO GET RESULTS   7
LAB WAIT TOO LONG   3
DON'T NOTIFY IF NML   2
PREFER LETTER ONLY   1

0   10   20   30   40   50
NUMBER OF TIMES

Some patients made more than 1 comment
Tally represents all comments made

(continued)

Quality-of-Care Measurement Laboratory Feedback Study
Executive Summary July 1991 (continued)

How Patients Were Informed of Their Test Results (%)

Health Center	A	B	C	D	E	F	G	H	I	Total
Patient Called	14.0	15.3	6.2	10.0	13.3	9.5	7.0	8.3	5.2	9.9
Clinician Called	9.0	17.0	19.0	7.8	20.0	12.4	9.5	15.0	11.5	12.5
Letter Sent	27.4	45.8	44.3	33.0	28.1	51.2	46.0	37.6	57.9	41.3
More Than 1 Method	29.5	11.4	28.0	22.7	18.6	10.1	23.7	26.0	16.8	20.7
Other	10.3	7.0	2.5	10.6	9.4	14.1	10.7	9.4	4.9	8.8
Not Notified	9.3	2.1	0	11.8	10.6	2.7	3.1	1.7	3.9	5.0
Missing	0	1.4	0	4.1	0	0	0	2.0	0	0.8

Overall Satisfaction with Method of Notification (%)

Health Center	A	B	C	D	E	F	G	H	I	Total
Excellent	25.6	17.5	28.2	14.7	32.8	27.0	21.3	36.2	25.6	22.9
Very Good	39.4	45.7	34.9	41.0	45.3	44.9	34.6	18.5	40.4	38.3
Good	18.3	29.1	21.0	33.6	12.0	20.4	19.2	14.4	20.7	21.5
Fair	11.0	12.4	7.2	6.2	7.8	6.7	10.9	15.9	10.1	9.8
Poor	4.5	5.3	6.7	2.3	2.1	1.0	10.0	7.6	3.2	4.7
Missing	1.2	0	2	2.4	0	0	4.0	2.4	0	1.3
%MAS*	67.9	69.5	65.4	62.4	74.8	72.6	56.0	58.4	69.2	64.6

*One hundred percent is, of course, the theoretical maximum achieveable score. To figure the Maximum Achieveable Score (MAS), each percentage point in the "excellent" category is given its full weight; the "very good" category is given 75% of its weight; "good," 50%; "fair," 25%; and "poor," 0%. The sum of all these is multiplied by the difference between 100% and the percentage points in the "missing" row.

How Patients Rated Each Method of Notification (%)

	EXCL	VRGD	GOOD	FAIR	POOR	MISSING
Patient Called	12.9	22.8	31.0	24.6	2.0	6.7
Clinician Called	47.9	32.1	10.3	6.2	2.5	1.0
Letter Sent	33.3	33.3	25.7	5.7	2.0	0
More Than 1 Method	39.5	24.8	23.9	10.2	1.6	0
Other	16.9	16.9	29.4	17.2	18.7	0.9
Not Notified	0	0	4.3	7.8	71.0	16.9
Missing	0	0	0	0	0	100

Summary Notes

- This annual QCM measurement determines: frequency of notification for normal results; distribution of methods used to notify; and patients' level of satisfaction associated with the notification process.
- Surveys mailed to patients who had a normal urinalysis, a normal blood test, and/or a normal Pap smear during Q3 & Q4 FY89.
- 1331 surveys mailed, 521 returned usable, representing 39.1% response rate.
- 93.5% of respondents were notified of their results.
- %MAS satisfaction rating for method of notification is 64.6% ("good" to "very good").

Figure 7.R. Quality-of-care summary on methods used by nine health centers (code named A-I) to notify patients of laboratory test results. The series of graphs and tables focuses attention on which methods of notification patients prefer and how this affects their satisfaciton with each health center. (Both the numerical and bar graph results presented are fictitious.)
Source: Harvard Community Health Plan, Brookline, MA, 1990. Used with permission.

Correlation Between Condition on Discharge and Neuroleptic Drug Dosage on Day 14

CONDITION ON DISCHARGE	THERAPEUTIC DOSAGE OF NEUROLEPTIC DRUG ON DAY 14		TOTAL
	Yes	**No**	
Improved or better	33	7	40
Unimproved or deteriorated	2	8	10
Total	35	15	50

Correlation Between Physician Category and Neuroleptic Drug Dosage on Day 14

CATEGORY OF PATIENT'S PHYSICIAN	THERAPEUTIC DOSAGE OF NEUROLEPTIC DRUG ON DAY 14		TOTAL
	Yes	**No**	
Salaried physician	24	1	25
Physician in private practice	11	14	25
Total	35	15	50

FIGURE 7.S. Often monitoring and evaluation data must be broken out in more than one way to highlight a trend of care. Taken together, these two tables suggest a correlation between drug dosage deficiencies and category of physician.

Repeat Films by Technologist and Discrepancy Type

Technologist:	Over-Exposed	Under-Exposed	Improper Position	Equipment Malfunction	Other	Total Repeats	% of Total Repeats
A	1		3			4	5.79
B	5	3	14		1	23	7.07
C	1		1			2	
D	2				4		8.73
E		4	13	1	1	19	8.87
F	1	1	1		1	4	
G	2	8	9		6	25	5.81
I	3	5	6	1	1	16	7.01
K	7	5	6		1	19	4.51
L	3	2	3		1	9	5.88
M	1	8	4	1	2	16	5.42
N	1					1	
O	5	4	2			11	7.58
P		2				2	
					Total		6.66

Examination Types with the Most Repeat Films, with Cause of Repeat

Part/Exam:	Improper Positioning	Incorrect Technique	Equipment Malfunction	Technologist Error	Total
Chest: PA	6	9	1		16
Lateral	3	4			7
AP	3	7			10
Decubitus		1			1
Tomo's: IVC	3	4		1	8
Gallbladder	1	1			2
Kidney	2	2			4
Chest	1				1
Shoulder				1	1
Lumbar Spine: AP	1	1			2
Lithotomy	1	2			3
Oblique	1	1			2
Lateral		1			1
L5-S1 Spot	6				6

(continued)

Examination Types with the Most Repeat Films, with Cause of Repeat (continued)

Part/Exam:	Improper Positioning	Incorrect Technique	Equipment Malfunction	Technologist Error	Total
Thoracic Spine: AP	2				2
Lateral		1			1
Spot T12		1			1
Skull: Townes	2	1			3
PA	2				2
Laws	3	1			4
Stenvers		1			1
Sinuses: Caldwell	4				4
Waters	1				1
Shoulder: AP		2			2
Axial	1	2			3
Abdomen: AP		7		1	8
Bladder	2				2
Femur: AP	2	3			5
Lateral		2			2
Accidental Film Advance:			4		4
Improper Fluoro. Technique:				7	7
Spot in Fluoro. Carriage:				5	5

PA = Posteroanterior or back-to-front; AP = Anteroposterior or front-to-back

Repeat Films by Discrepancy Type and Room

Room Number	Over-Exposed	Under-Exposed	Improper Positioning	Equipment Malfunction	Other	Totals
ROOM #2	5	5	12			22
ROOM #3	5	3	1			9
ROOM #4	12	19	32		1	64
ROOM #5	1	6	7		4	18
ROOM #6	2	5	3	4		14
ROOM #7	1	1			1	3
ROOM #8		3	10		11	24
ROOM #9	3	7	8		2	20
PORTABLES	2	4	2			8
						182

FIGURE 7.T. *Three tables show how indicator data was grouped to find causes underlying radiology film repeats. Among other things, the data suggest a need for further investigation of PA (posteroanterior or back-to-front) chest exams and of exams performed in room #4.*
SOURCE: *Adapted from Department of Radiology, Good Samaritan Medical Center, Lutheran Hospital Campus, Milwaukee. Used with permission.*

Data Collected on Scheduling Problems in 200 Cases

Clinician	Number of Cases in Study	First Treatment Session				Subsequent Treatment Sessions		All Treatment Sessions			
		Scheduled Within Three-Day Period		Seen Within Three-Day Period		Scheduled Appointment Exceeded Ten-Day Interval		Client Resistance Noted		No Shows	
		Number	%	Number	%	Number	%	Number	%	Number	%
1	20	12	60	8	40	12	60	2	10	5	25
2	18	11	61	8	44	3	17	0	0	2	11
3	26	12	46	9	35	14	54	4	15	10	38
4	17	14	82	8	47	4	24	0	0	5	29
5	21	14	67	8	38	6	29	4	19	8	38
6	20	14	70	8	40	6	30	1	5	2	10
7	12	12	100	8	67	1	8	0	0	0	0
8	28	10	36	7	25	20	71	6	21	14	50
9	19	14	74	8	42	0	0	3	16	5	26
10	19	15	79	8	42	0	0	0	0	2	11
Total	200	128	64	80	40	66	33	20	10	53	27

Treatment Sessions Scheduled to Occur Within Three Days of Initial Contact

Occurrence of Treatment Session Within Three Days of Contact	Percentage of No Shows
Yes	6
No	17

Day of Week of Initial Contact and Number of Treatment Sessions Scheduled to Occur Within Three Days

		M	T	W	T	F	S	S	Total
Number of Initial Contacts		25	25	20	22	40	36	32	200
Initial Treatment Session Scheduled to Occur Within Three Days	Number	22	23	15	10	16	24	18	128
	Percentage	88	92	75	45	40	67	56	64

(continued)

Day of Week of Initial Contact and Number of Treatment Sessions Occurring Within Three Days (continued)

		M	T	W	T	F	S	S	Total
NUMBER OF INITIAL CONTACTS		25	25	20	22	40	36	32	200
OCCURRENCE OF TREATMENT SESSION WITHIN THREE DAYS	NUMBER	18	20	6	8	8	14	6	80
	PERCENTAGE	72	80	30	36	20	39	19	40

Number of Completed Sessions Prior to No Show

COMPLETED SESSIONS PRIOR TO NO SHOWS	0	1	2	3	4	5	6	7	8	9	10+
NO SHOWS	26	6	6	4	4	3	0	2	0	1	1

Intervals Between Treatment Sessions in Relation to No Shows for 27 Clients Who Completed at Least One Session

INTERVALS BETWEEN TREATMENT SESSIONS	NUMBER OF NO SHOWS	PERCENTAGE OF NO SHOWS
More than ten days	20	74
Ten days or less	7	26

FIGURE 7.U. *Example of how data can be broken out by multiple parameters to find patterns in care associated with appointment scheduling problems. For example, the high rate of "no shows" appears linked to certain clinicians, days of the week, number of completed sessions prior to the no show, and intervals between treatment sessions.*

Room Turnover Times

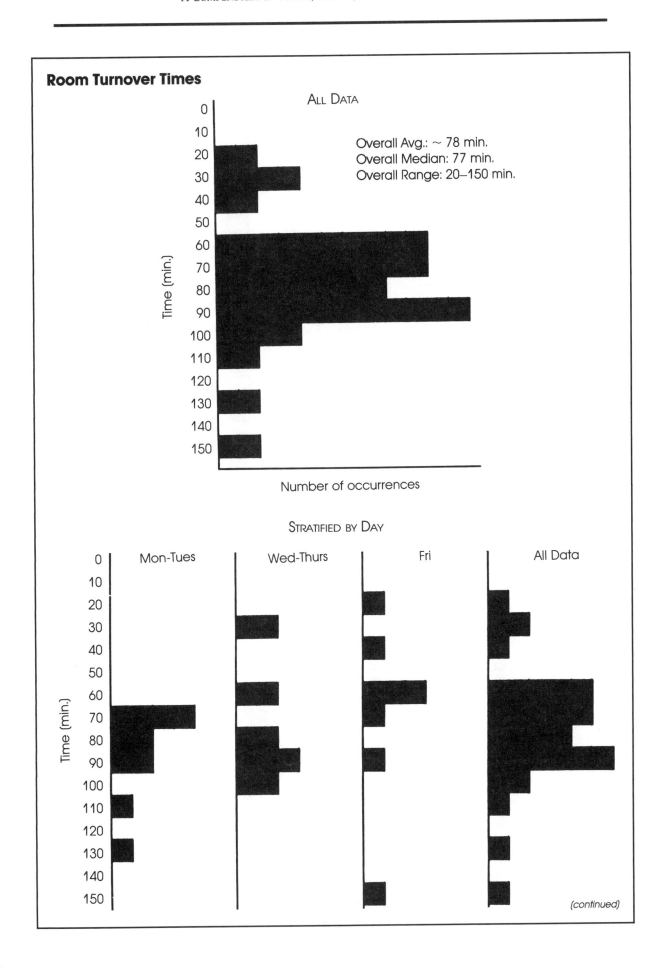

Overall Avg.: ~ 78 min.
Overall Median: 77 min.
Overall Range: 20–150 min.

(continued)

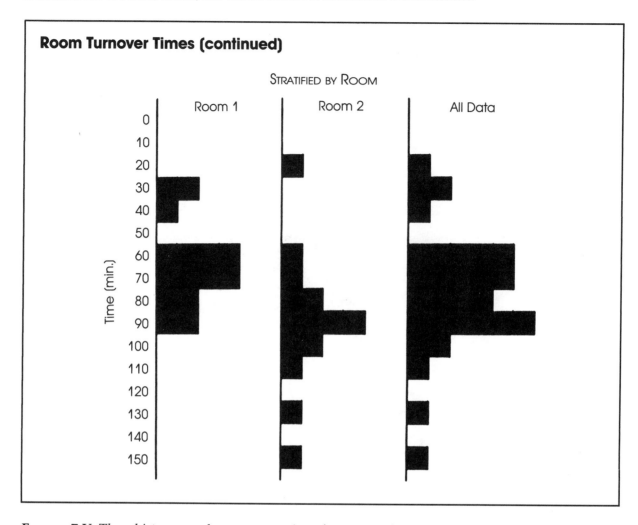

FIGURE 7.V. *Three histograms show turnover times for an open heart surgery suite. The second and third sections stratify turnover times by room and days of the week. Turnover times appear to be lower in Room 1 and on Friday.*
SOURCE: *Reprinted with permission from the National Demonstration Project on Quality Improvement in Health Care, a project of Harvard Community Health Plan and the John A. Hartford Foundation, Brookline, MA.*

What Causes A Complication?

WHAT CAUSES A COMPLICATION?

PHYSICIAN/ TECHNIQUE

Training

Learning curve

Supervision

Approach

MATERIALS

Multiple vendors

No kits

Break easily

Kits missing supplies

COMPLICATIONS

Beds

"Code 99"

"Redo"

Lighting

Unstable during procedure

Can't pull away from wall

Can't adjust height

Time of Day

No RNs at night

No supervision at night

When to measure

Who measures

Definition of "CNS event"

X-Ray diagnosis of PTX

ENVIRONMENT

MEASUREMENTS

COMPLICATION RATE BY TIME OF DAY

Complication rate

15					
12					
9					
6					
3					
0					

(551) (355) (271) (147) (41) (48)

7-11A   11-3P   3-7P   7-11P   11-3A   3-7A

Total # of procedures

(continued)

What Causes A Complication? (continued)

NURSING COVERAGE DURING THE PLACEMENT OF CV & PA CATHETERS

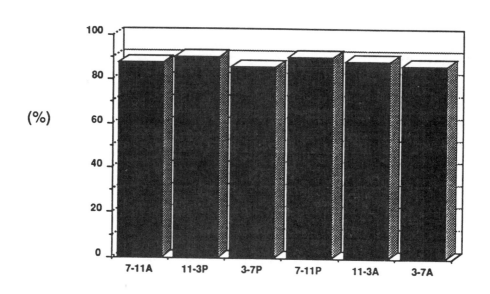

WHEN LINES ARE PLACED

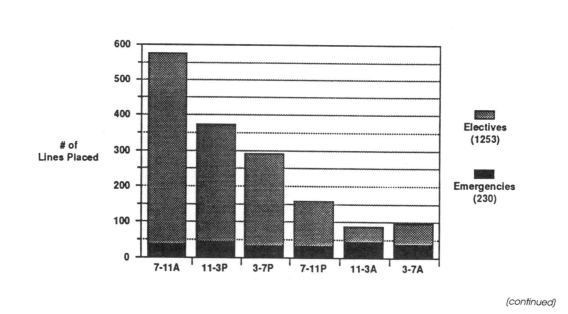

(continued)

What Causes A Complication? (continued)

COMPLICATION RATES

Electives	3.1	(39/1253)
Emergencies	15.2	(35/230)

COMPLICATION RATES IN ELECTIVE CASES
BY ACCESS SITE

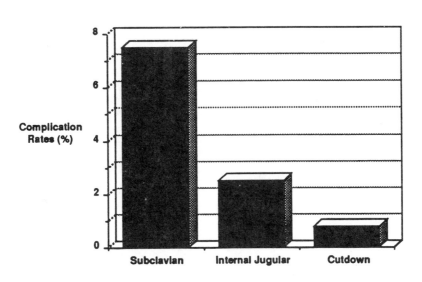

(continued)

What Causes A Complication? (continued)

COMPLICATION RATES IN ELECTIVE CASES BY SITE OF PROCEDURE

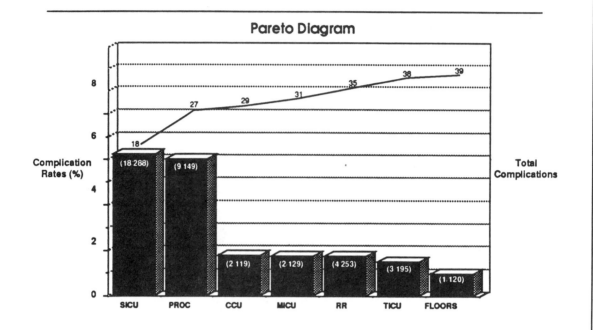

COMPLICATION RATES IN ELECTIVE CASES: ACCESS SITE VARY BY SITE OF PROCEDURE

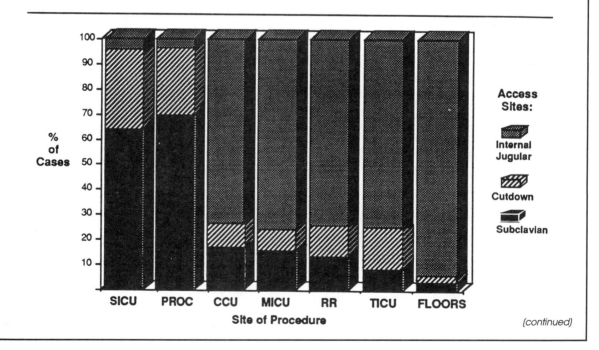

(continued)

What Causes A Complication? (continued)

COMPLICATION RATES IN EMERGENCY CASES WHY ARE THEY HIGHER?

Uncontrollable Causes

Hypotension

Code situation

Controllable Causes

MDs use different kits

COMPLICATION RATES IN EMERGENCY CASES DEPARTMENTS STOCK DIFFERENT CATHETERS

Departments	Companies
Surgery	Manufacturer A
Medicine	Manufacturer B
Anesthesia	Manufacturer C

COMPLICATION RATES IN EMERGENCY CASES STRATIFIED BY DEPARTMENT AND CATHETER

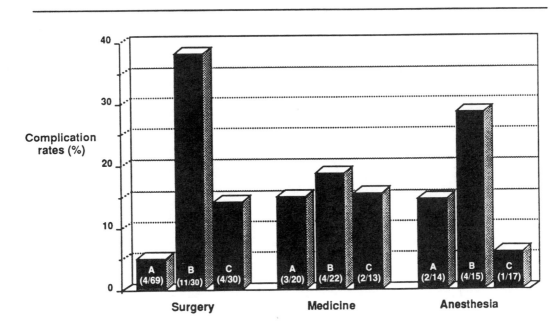

(continued)

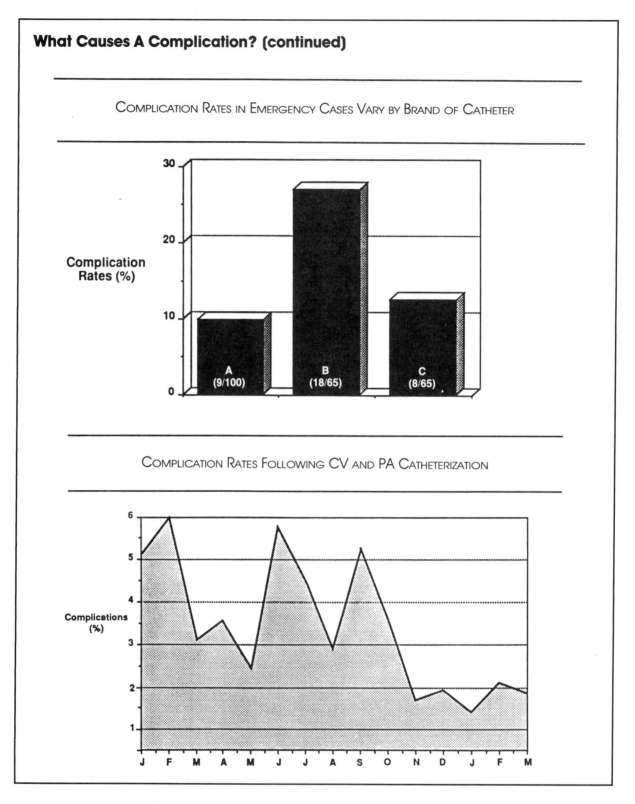

FIGURE 7.W. *A series of 14 graphs and tables showing an evaluation into a high complication rate after placement of CVP and PA catheters. Problems were traced to brand of catheters access sites, and sites of procedure. Many of these graphic tools are those often used in a continuous quality improvement model. See Figures 7.KK. through 7.RR. for more on these models.*
SOURCE: *Reprinted with permission from the National Demonstration Project on Quality Improvement in Health Care, a project of Harvard Community Health Plan and the John A. Hartford Foundation, Brookline, MA.*

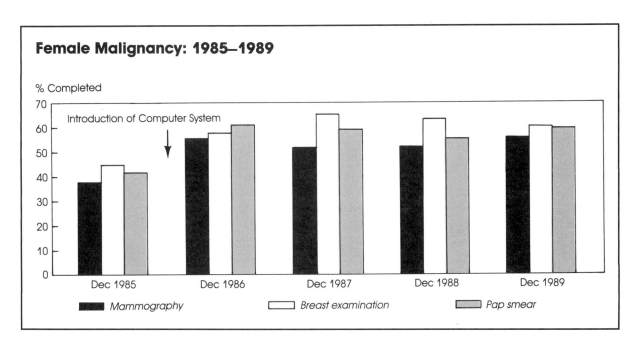

Figure 7.X. *This chart highlights desired improvement in the percentage of completed female malignancy screenings after action was taken to improve care. A series of bar charts can show trends in occurrence rates of several indicators over time.*
Source: *Chodroff CH: Cancer screening and immunization quality assurance using a personal computer. QRB 16(8):286, Aug 1990.*

Summary Pediatric Hospital Evaluation: 1990

Purpose: To assess pediatricians' perceptions of quality at hospitals they use. Results for Hospital A and Hospital B are summarized below.

High (> = 80% MAS) 1990 ratings	A	B	Low (< = 50% MAS) 1990 ratings	A	B
Avail. of ICU and non-ICU beds	X	X	Avail. of x-ray/lab during hosp.	X	X
Qual. of house staff & nursing care	X		Avail. of x-ray/lab posthosp.	X	
Qual. of ES physician staff	X	X	Avail. of old hospital chart		X
Relationship: Gastroent. & Gen. Surg.		X	Integration of amb./hosp. records	X	X
Appropriate care level	X		Relationship with Cardio. & Ortho.		X
Ease of arranging outpatient ES		X	Parking arrangements	X	X
Ability to arrange prompt discharge	X		Cost of care	X	
Convenience of rounding	X				
Relationship: Urology, Gen. Surg. Ophthalmology & Cardio-thoracic	X				

TRENDS OVER TIME:

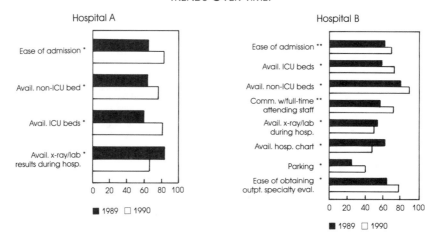

*Noteworthy difference, 1989-1990, p < .05; ** Significant difference, p < .01.*

CORRELATES OF SATISFACTION:

Familiarity with hospital correlated significantly with satisfaction:

More hospital experience → LOWER satisfaction on:

- ease of obtaining x-ray/lab results in hospital
- relationship with ES, Infectious Disease
- availability of old hospital chart
- quality of nursing/house staff care
- convenience of cover rounds

More hospital experience → HIGHER satisfaction on:

- communication with full-time attending staff
- availability of old hospital chart
- quality of nursing care
- control management of patient
- ability to arrange discharge
- ease of obtaining social service
- cost of care

CONCLUSIONS:

- Significant improvements at Hospital A on admitting, access to information, and communication with full-time attending staff
- Significant improvement on admitting at Hospital B
- Other Hospitals: At Hospital C inpatient diagnostic intensity and relationship with ES remain low; At Hospital D, ES and outpatient evaluation rated low.

FIGURE 7.Y. An HMO uses this report to compare its satisfaction with two area hospitals to which it refers patients. Paired bars show changes over time in satisfaction with each hospital. (The satisfaction findings presented are entirely fictitious.)
SOURCE: Harvard Community Health Plan, Brookline, MA, 1990. Used with permission.

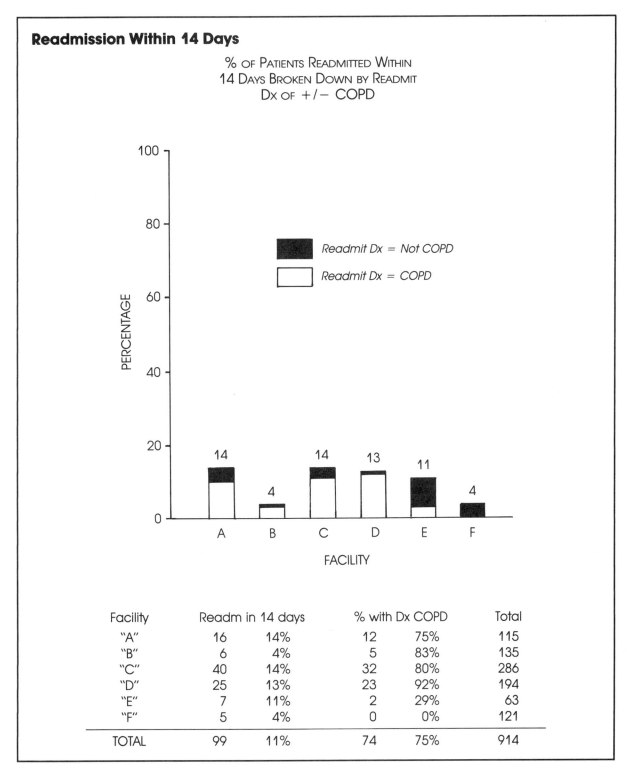

Readmission Within 14 Days

% OF PATIENTS READMITTED WITHIN
14 DAYS BROKEN DOWN BY READMIT
DX OF +/− COPD

Legend:
- ■ Readmit Dx = Not COPD
- □ Readmit Dx = COPD

(Y-axis: PERCENTAGE; X-axis: FACILITY, values A B C D E F)

Bar labels: A = 14, B = 4, C = 14, D = 13, E = 11, F = 4

Facility	Readm in 14 days		% with Dx COPD		Total
"A"	16	14%	12	75%	115
"B"	6	4%	5	83%	135
"C"	40	14%	32	80%	286
"D"	25	13%	23	92%	194
"E"	7	11%	2	29%	63
"F"	5	4%	0	0%	121
TOTAL	99	11%	74	75%	914

FIGURE 7.Z. *Graphs such as this can help make clear what may be contributing most to a pattern in care—in this case, patients with a diagnosis of chronic obstructive pulmonary disease (COPD) seem especially linked to a pattern of readmission within 14 days at facilities A, C, and D.*
SOURCE: *Chandler J, Tarver R: The care of the veteran with a diagnosis of COPD: A focused review of medical practice patterns in six VA facilities.* Journal of Quality Assurance 11(6):10, Dec/Jan 1989-1990.

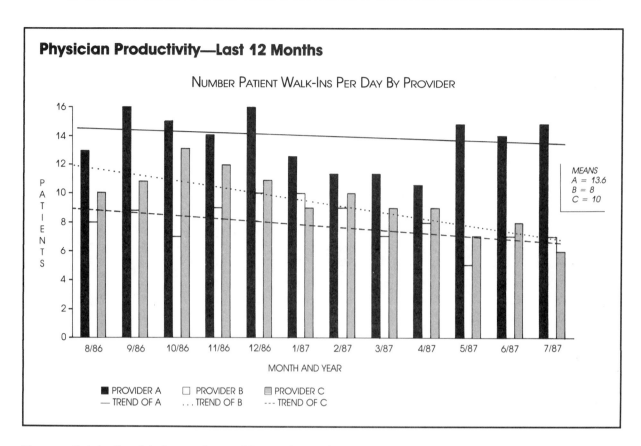

Figure 7.AA. *Graphic format for tracking patient volume among multiple practitioners.*
Source: *Veterans Administration Outpatient Clinic, Worchester, MA. Used with permission.*

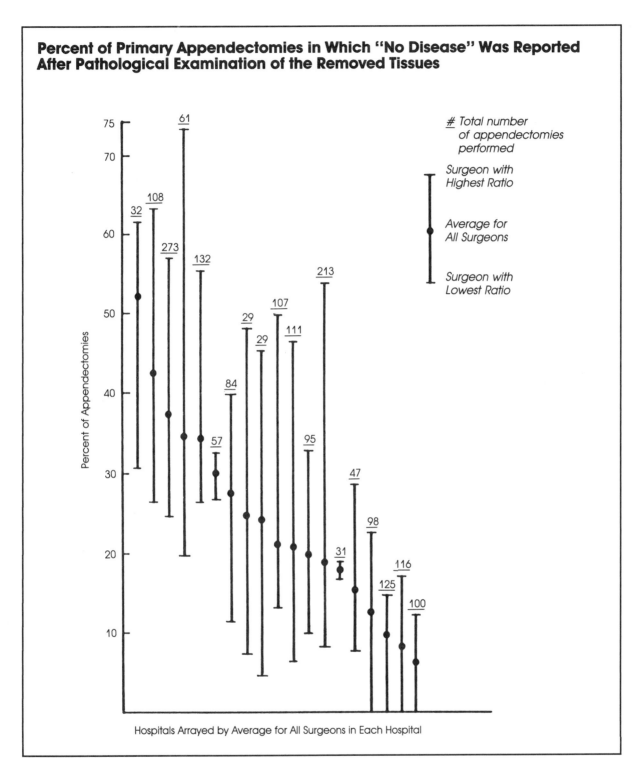

FIGURE 7.BB. Chart shows average performance as well as range in an easy-to-grasp format.
SOURCE: Adapted from Weeks HA: Tightness of Organization Related to Patterns of Patient Care.
Bureau of Public Health Economics, School of Public Health, University of Michigan. (Adapted in
Donabedian A: Explorations in Quality Assessment and Monitoring, Vol III, The Methods and
Findings of Quality Assessment and Monitoring: An Illustrated Analysis. *Ann Arbor, MI:*
Health Administration Press, 1985, p 139).

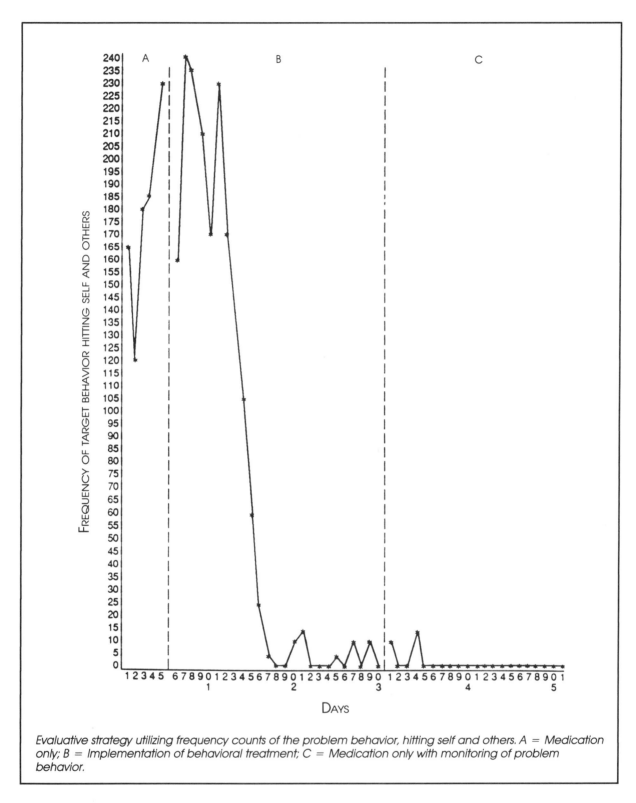

Evaluative strategy utilizing frequency counts of the problem behavior, hitting self and others. A = Medication only; B = Implementation of behavioral treatment; C = Medication only with monitoring of problem behavior.

FIGURE 7.CC. *Three line graphs showing relative improvement brought by three actions to improve care. The evaluation strategy here utilized frequency counts of the problem behavior, hitting self and others.*
SOURCE: *Desch JR: Quality assurance as an information system for an era of increasing accountability.* Topics in Health Record Management 10(2):33-44, Dec 1989.

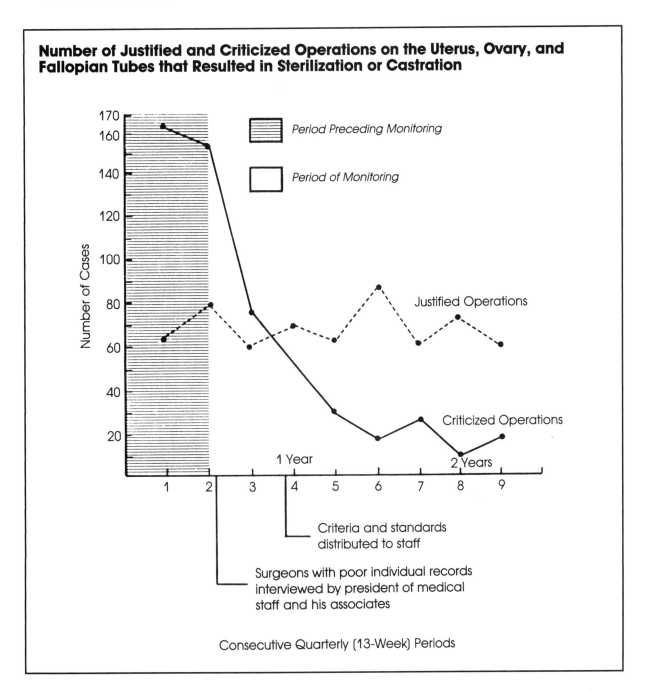

FIGURE 7.DD. *Line graphs such as this can illustrate improvement resulting from monitoring and evaluation actions.*
SOURCE: *Adapted from Lembcke, PA: Medical auditing by scientific methods: Illustrated by major female pelvic surgery.* JAMA, *162:653, October 13, 1956 (adapted in Donabedian A:* Explorations in Quality Assessment and Monitoring, Vol III, The Methods and Findings of Quality Assessment and Monitoring: An Illustrated Analysis. *Ann Arbor, MI: Health Administration Press, 1985, p 145).*

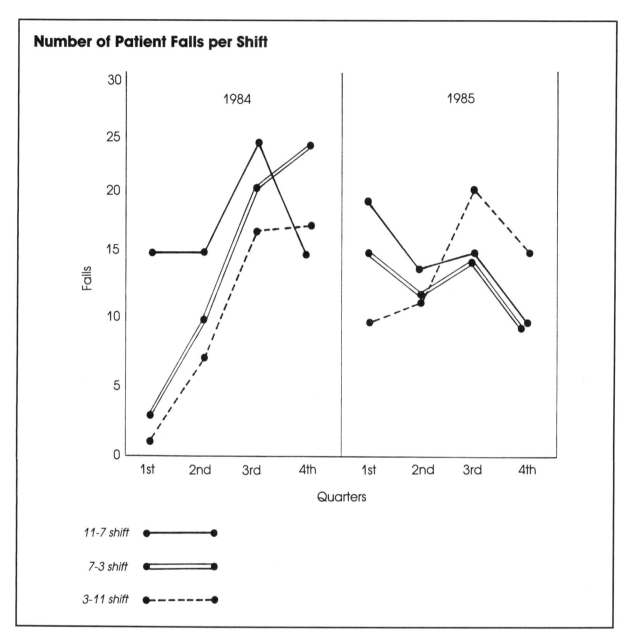

FIGURE 7.EE. *Example of how to use multiple line graphs when illustrating trends in monitoring data.*

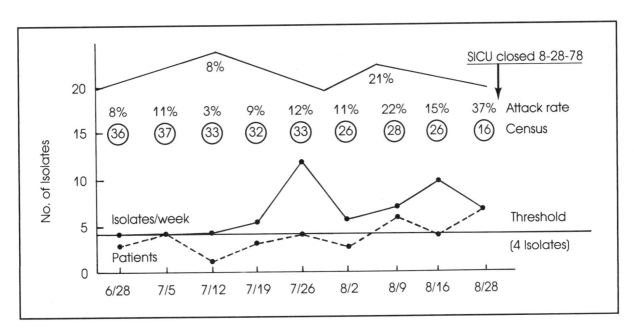

FIGURE 7.FF. *An example of the large amount of information a line graph and accompanying data can convey. This is a graph of data gathered for "bug surveillance" before and during a Pseudomonas outbreak in a surgical intensive care unit (SICU). The threshold value had been set at four isolates for this organism. The heavy solid line represents the number of infected patients each week during a nine-week period. The circled figures (census) above the plotted lines indicate the number of patients treated in the SICU (that is, the number of patients exposed to the organism), and the percentages (attack rate) indicate ratios of the numbers of infected patients to those exposed each week. The percentages at the top of the figure—8% and 21%—are averages of the attack rate preceding and during the outbreak. Investigation of this infection problem led to temporary closing of the SICU for a thorough cleaning.* **SOURCE:** *McGuckin MB: An innovative approach to surveillance of nosocomial outbreaks. QRB 1979 Special Edition, p 37.*

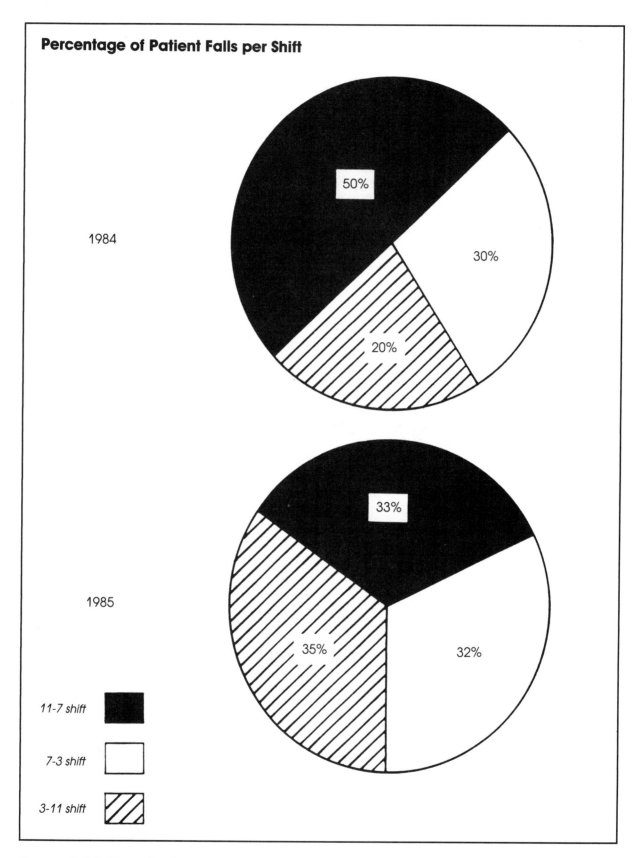

FIGURE 7.GG. *Example of a pie graph. Pie graphs can be used to display data such as factors that were associated with or contributed to a variation discovered through monitoring and evaluation.*

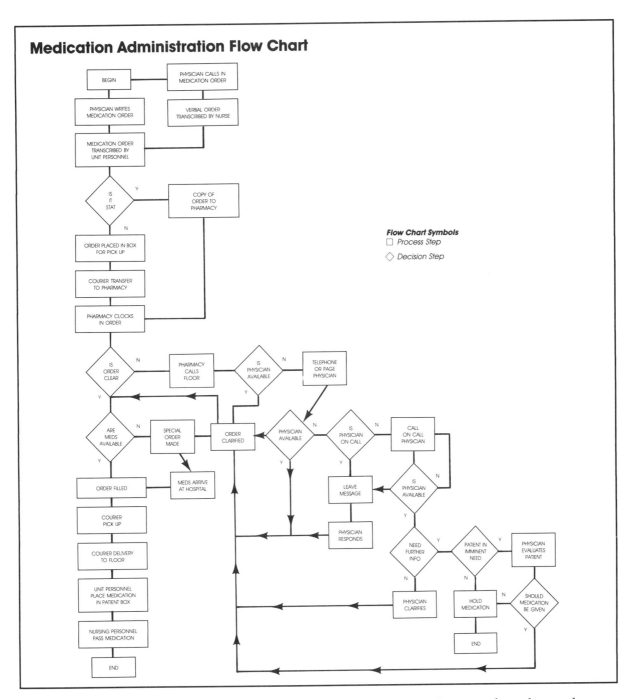

Medication Administration Flow Chart

Flow Chart Symbols
☐ Process Step
◇ Decision Step

Figure 7.HH. Process *flowcharts are representations of the sequence of steps performed to produce a specific output. "The easiest and best way to understand a process is to draw a picture of it—that's basically what flowcharting is," writes John T. Burr.* The idea behind a flowchart is that a process cannot be improved unless everyone understands and agrees on what the process is. After delineating the current process, staff should be able to identify redundancies, inefficiencies, and misunderstandings, and also streamline and improve processes.*

One way to proceed is to create two charts: one on the sequence of steps to be taken if everything worked right and another that charts the steps the process actually *follows. The people who have the greatest knowledge of the process being examined must be involved in making the chart; this should include those who actually perform the work that sustains the process.*

Source: HCA West Paces Ferry Hospital, Atlanta. Used with permission.

*Burr JT: The tools of quality, Part 1: Going with the flow(chart). Quality Progress 23(6):64, *June 1990.*

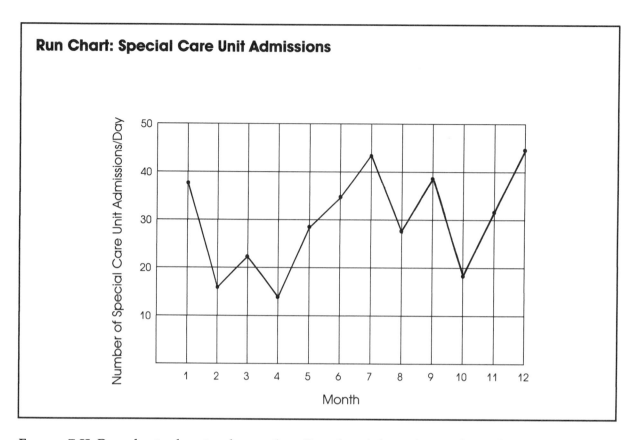

Run Chart: Special Care Unit Admissions

Figure 7.II. Run charts *show trends over time. Run chart information can be used to evaluate the effect of actions to improve care processes. As an example, "when nine points 'run' on one side of the average it indicates a statistically unusual event and that the average has changed," according to* The Memory Jogger: A Pocket Guide of Tools for Continuous Improvement. *"Such changes should always be investigated. If the shift is favorable, it should be made a permanent part of the system. If it is unfavorable, it should be eliminated."*
Source: Brassard M: The Memory Jogger: A Pocket Guide of Tools for Continuous Improvement, *2nd ed, Methuen, MA: Goal/QPC, 1988, p 31.*

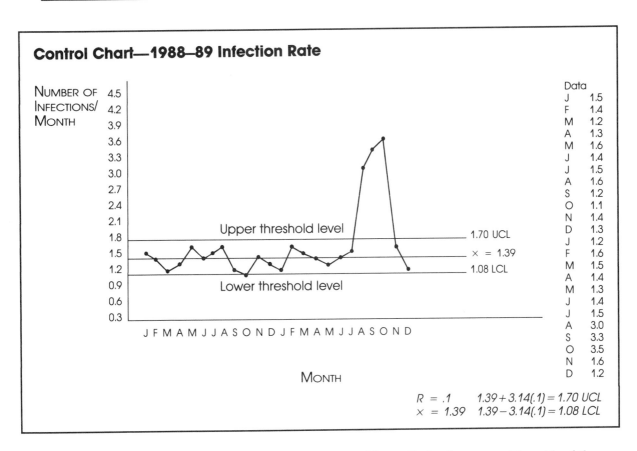

Control Chart—1988–89 Infection Rate

							Data	
Number of Infections/ Month	4.5						J	1.5
	4.2						F	1.4
	3.9						M	1.2
	3.6						A	1.3
	3.3						M	1.6
	3.0						J	1.4
	2.7						J	1.5
	2.4						A	1.6
	2.1		Upper threshold level			1.70 UCL	S	1.2
	1.8						O	1.1
	1.5					x = 1.39	N	1.4
	1.2					1.08 LCL	D	1.3
	0.9		Lower threshold level				J	1.2
	0.6						F	1.6
	0.3						M	1.5
							A	1.4
							M	1.3
							J	1.4
							J	1.5
		J F M A M J J A S O N D J F M A M J J A S O N D					A	3.0
							S	3.3
							O	3.5
							N	1.6
		Month					D	1.2

$$R = .1 \qquad 1.39 + 3.14(.1) = 1.70 \; UCL$$
$$x = 1.39 \qquad 1.39 - 3.14(.1) = 1.08 \; LCL$$

Figure 7.JJ. A control chart *is a run chart with upper and lower limits drawn on either side of the process average. The upper and lower control limits are determined by allowing a process to run untouched and then calculating the standard deviation of variation in the indicator data being monitored. Often, as in this figure, two standard deviations may be used as control limits. (In a normal distribution, only 1 in 20 rates will differ from the mean by more than twice the standard deviation.) This chart is filled out with hypothetical rates and is not based on real data.*

Control charts are tools for distinguishing between variations in a process that are inherent (eg, because of poor process design) and those that are intermittent and/or unpredictable (eg, equipment failure). They are also useful in determing an indicator's threshold for evaluation, as indicated in Figure 5.B. and discussed at length in Appendix C, p 279. For explanation on how to construct and use control charts see Appendix C.

Source: *Developed by Linda Owen, Quality Assurance Specialist; Judith Quirt, Coordinator, Infection Control Program; Carl Weston, MD, Vice-President, Medical Affairs; and Mary Zimmerman, Director, Quality Resources from Meriter Hospital, Inc, Madison, WI, 1990. Used with permission.*

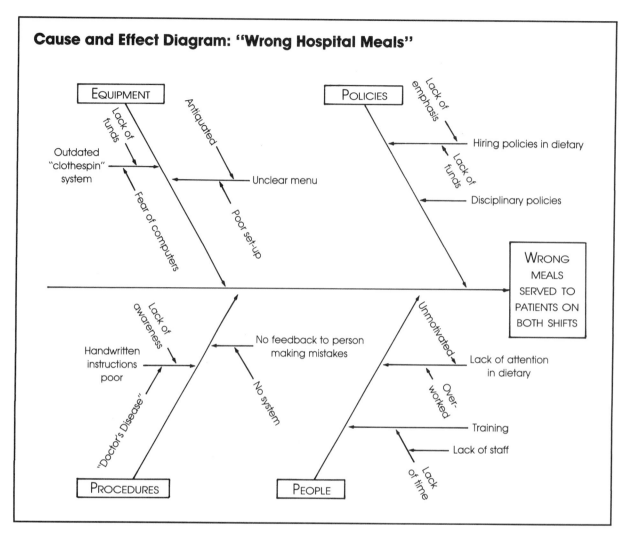

FIGURE 7.KK. *The* cause-and-effect diagram *is a tool for obtaining information about processes and their output. Through construction of these diagrams (also called fishbone or Ishikawa diagrams), possible causes of a specific problem or condition are explored and displayed. Brainstorming can be used to identify possible causes, which can be grouped around four basic categories: materials, methods, manpower, and machines. The effect or symptom being examined is placed at the right, enclosed in a box. The process of creating a cause-and-effect diagram is educational. When developed by a team (as it should be), it promotes discussion and evaluation of an assortment of perspectives.*
Source: The Memory Jogger: A Pocket Guide of Tools for Continuous Improvement, *1st ed,* Methuen, MA: Goal/QPC.

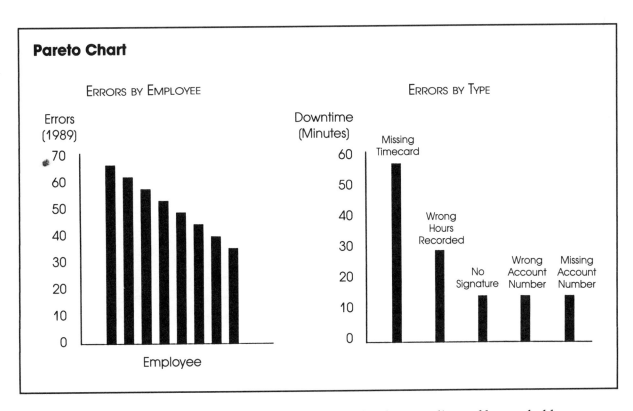

FIGURE 7.LL. A Pareto chart *is a comparison of factors related to a quality problem ranked by frequency of occurrence. (The most frequently occuring event is represented at the far left, with other events represented to the right in descending order.) It is a tool for fact-based priority setting, used to sort out the "vital few" factors or causes related to a quality problem from the "trivial many" (ie, the 80/20 principle). This type of vertical bar graph is used to help determine which problems to solve in which order.*

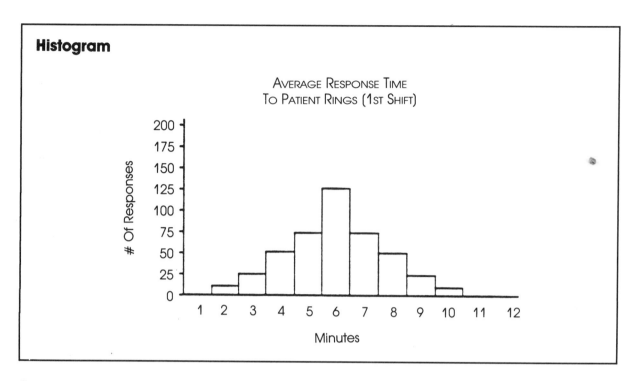

FIGURE 7.MM. *A* histogram *is a graphic summary of the pattern of variation in a set of data. The pictorial nature of the histogram makes patterns apparent that would be difficult to see in a simple table of numbers. The creator of the histogram is looking for surprise variations in the distribution that signal potential problems. While these are vertical graphs like Pareto charts, they differ in that they display the distribution of data rather than the characteristics of a product or service. Since all repeated events produce results that vary over time, histograms reveal the amount of variation that a process has within it.*
SOURCE: *Brassard M:* The Memory Jogger: A Pocket Guide of Tools for Continuous Improvement, *2nd ed, Methuen, MA: Goal/QPC, 1988, p 42.*

Check Sheet

Errors	Jan	Feb	Mar	Apr	May	Jun	Jul	Aug	Sep	Oct	Total
Type 1	////	//	//	////	////	//			~~HHT~~ /	~~HHT~~ ////	33
Type 2			//		///	//	////	//			13
Type 3	/	/	///		////	~~HHT~~ /	/		~~HHT~~ /	~~HHT~~ ////	31
Type 4					////		///			~~HHT~~ ///	15
Type 5			/					/			2
Type 6											0
Type 7									/	///	4
Total	5	3	8	4	15	10	8	3	13	29	98

Figure 7.NN. A check sheet *is a simple data recording form designed to provide answers to the question, "How often are certain events happening?" It is used to gather data based on observations of how often certain events occur (eg, errors per day of the week, per product, per staff member, and by type of error). As a way to collect data, it could also be included under Step 6 of this book, which addresses data collection and organization.*

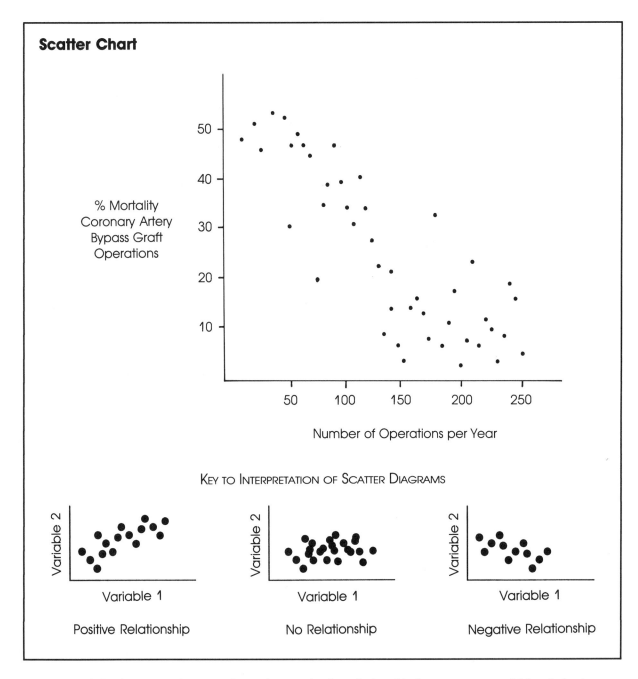

FIGURE 7.OO. *A scatter diagram is used to study the relationship between two variables, bringing up possible cause-and-effect relationships. Paired data is plotted. A scatter diagram might be used to chart the relationship between a worker's training and number of errors or between light levels and computer errors. The direction and "tightness" of the dot cluster gives a clue as to the strength of the relationship between the two variables (see inset for examples of this).*
SOURCE: *Merry MD: Total quality management for physicians: Translating the new paradigm. QRB 16(3):103, Mar 1990. Used with permission.*

The Evaluation Process

IMPORTANT ASPECT OF CARE:

INDICATOR:

THRESHOLD FOR EVALUATION:

OPPORTUNITY FOR IMPROVEMENT/PROBLEM (description and date identified):

DEPARTMENTS/SERVICES/COMMITTEES/PERSONS INVOLVED:

NOTE PATIENT CARE TRENDS ISOLATED THROUGH EVALUATION:

WHAT TYPES OF DATA WERE TRENDED:

What data was not available?

Are there plans to collect this data? Yes _____ No _____

When _____

Plan for data collection:

WILL FURTHER EVALUATION BE CONDUCTED? WHY OR WHY NOT?

PLAN AND SCHEDULE OF FURTHER EVALUATION:

RECOMMENDATIONS/ACTION TAKEN

(If action is to be taken, state activity, by whom, and when):

FOLLOW-UP MONITORING/ACTIONS:

DEPARTMENT DIRECTOR/DIRECTOR OF NURSING _____

DATE: _____

QA DEPARTMENT _____

DATE: _____

FIGURE 7.PP. Form designed to help document the evaluation process.

Deficiency Analysis Question Guide

	Attribution	Yes/No	Comments/Analysis
1. Are provider recruitment, screening, hiring, orientation, and initial training programs inadequate or inefficient? 2. Are in-service training and continuing education programs inadequate or inefficient?	Administration		Inadequate policies or procedures
3. Was the chain of command misunderstood? Are job descriptions and responsibilities unclear? Do providers lack sufficient authority to execute their responsibilities? Are divided responsibilities causing confusion? Is support staff improperly supervised? 4. Are there nonproductive and insufficient staff meetings, conferences, interdisciplinary and shift-to-shift communications?			
5. Are there planning difficulties? Confused priorities? Unmet deadlines?			Lack of personnel
6. Is there inefficient or uneven distribution of responsibilities of providers? 7. Does the facility lack, or lack access to, important services (ie, dietitian, social service, or rehabilitation department)? Are necessary services available but inadequate?			
8. Is equipment inadequate and insufficient? Outdated? Improperly maintained?			Lack of equipment
9. Are general recordkeeping systems inefficient and unresponsive to needs?			Inadequate medical record forms
10. Are insufficient time and inadequate space factors?			Environment
11. Was equipment not used because of inconvenient access?			
12. Are hospital policies or standard procedures not being enforced?			Knew, did not do
13. Is the facility's public relations program to explain the work of the institution and its service to the community and to enlist community support ineffective? Nonexistent? 14. Is the facility's volunteer program ineffective? Nonexistent? 15. Are patients unable to verbalize an understanding of their illness, home or follow-up care due to communication problems (eg, lack of translator for foreign-language-speaking patient)?			Inadequate hospital policies and procedures

(continued)

Deficiency Analysis Question Guide (continued)

	Attribution	Yes/No	Comments/Analysis
16. Are administrative tasks not performed for other reasons? Were inappropriate providers given the responsibility for treatment and approaches?	Administration (continued)		Knew, did not do
17. Is there evidence that staff did not have sufficient information? Knowledge? Skill? Training?	Staff		Lack of knowledge or skills

18. Were the approaches (ie, orders, treatments, procedures, services) improperly performed? Were there instances of neglect? Mistakes? Inconsistency or irregularity of care?
 	
19. If the responsible providers have demonstrated knowledge or skill, yet performance was inadequate, should motivational factors be considered?
 	
   A. Were providers unaware of the importance of the task?
   B. Were the tasks seemingly trivial? Punishing? Boring?
   C. Did providers lack in-group support and positive feedback?
   D. Were personal qualitites or personal problems involved?
   E. Was poor esprit de corps a factor?
			Knew, did not do

20. Was information inadequately documented because of provider unawareness of importance of charting?			Lack of documentation
21. Did patients receive unnecessary hospital and provider services?			Overutilization
22. Is there high turnover or poor morale among providers?			Other
23. Is there inadequate funding to meet patient's needs? 24. Are there local or state regulations that do not adequately consider patients' needs? 25. Are community support services lacking?	Community		Inadequate community resources
26. Are patients unable to verbalize and understand their illness, home or follow-up care due to their lack of understanding or intelligence? Was the patient's guardian (or significant other) excluded from the patient's education sessions?			Lack of knowledge or skill
27. Were any indicators found to be inadequate during variation analysis?	Other		Invalid screening criteria

Figure 7.QQ. *Questionnaire to help analyze variations in care or services. The questions raise issues possibly suggesting opportunities for improvement.*
Source: *Adapted from Fox L, Stearns G, Imbiorski W:* The Masters Manual for the Advanced Training of Hospital Audit Specialists. *Chicago: Care Communications, 1977, pp 142-146.*

Design Solutions and Controls

	| | | | | | | |							

PROPOSED SOLUTIONS

CRITERIA	Patient Test Reminder Systems	Patient Registry	Algorithm Reminder Systems	Clinician Education	Change Dx Test	Patient Education	"Same Day" Dx Testing	Test Tracing System
Technically Feasible	✔	✔	✔	✔	✔	✔		✔
Administratively Feasible	✔	✔	✔			✔		✔
Medically/Legally Feasible	✔	✔	✔	✔	✔	✔	✔	✔
Medically Acceptable	✔	✔	✔	✔	✔	✔	✔	✔
Reasonable Cost	✔	✔	✔			✔	✔	✔
Acceptable to Clinicians	✔	✔	✔			✔	✔	✔
Acceptable to Patients	✔	✔	✔	✔	✔	✔		✔
Likely to be Effective	✔	✔	✔				✔	✔

FIGURE 7.RR. *Matrix for assessing proposed solutions to a problem (horizontal axis) against several criteria (vertical axis).*
Source: *Reprinted with permission from the National Demonstration Project on Quality Improvement in Health Care, a project of Harvard Community Health Plan and the John A. Hartford Foundation, Brookline, Massachusetts.*

Questioned Trends/Incidents Spreadsheet

Dept/Indicator
Internal Medicine Monitors
Readmissions within 7 days
Month/Year   May 1988

Denominator Data		
Physician	Ttl Cases	Ttl Abstracted
(Code #s)		
1	3	
2	7	
3	2	
4	21	
5	11	

Total Questioned ___1___

• Ask why
• Evaluate the answer

(Continue on additional pages if necessary.)

Physician (Code)	Pt Record # (Code)	The Question and Relevant Findings	Physician Analyst/Dept Chmn Reaction					
			1*	2*	3*	4*	5*	"Because" + Reason
1	1	Patient readmitted with myocardial infarction 24 hours after discharge. Previous admission for "evaluation of chest pain"; no stress test ordered.			⊗			Because evaluation of chest pain was inadequate during the first admission.

*1 = Expected and acceptable. Reviewer comfortable.
*2 = Reasonable clinical controversy. Not totally unexpected. Reviewer still comfortable.
*3 = Very controversial. Unexpected. Reviewer uncomfortable.
*4 = Unexpected and unacceptable. Reviewer displeased.
*5 = Trend or incident requires formal corrective action.

Note to Physician Analyst: Make your judgment pretending you're the patient.

Figure 7.SS. Questioned trends and incidents spreadsheet designed to record peer review judgments.
Source: Thompson RE: The Hospitalwide Accountability System: Next Steps in Implementing Quality Improvement, *2nd ed. Wheaton, IL: SENSS Publications, 1990, p 58.*

Occurrence Screening Checklist

Severity Code (assign code to each confirmed APO) 0 = no injury 3 = major temporary 1 = minor temporary 4 = major permanent 2 = minor permanent 5 = death	Quality of Care Code (assign code to each confirmed APO) A - Standard of care met B - Standard of care questionable C - Standard of care not met

Physician Provider	( ) Concurrent Review ( ) Retrospective Review

Hospital Butler VAMC	Patient Name & SSN	Screener	Date	2nd Screener	Date

| Criteria   Element
No. | Occurrence found | | APO confirmed
2nd reviewer | Referred to
& date | APO confirmed
peer reviewer | Severity
code | Quality
code |
	Yes	Date					
1. Readmission within 14 days to an acute care bed							
2. Admission for adverse result or complication of outpatient care, nursing home care, or ambulatory surgery							
3. Unexpected transfer to special care unit from any other level care							
4. Unplanned return to the OR on this admission							
5. Unplanned removal, partial removal, injury, or repair of normal organ or structure during operative procedure							
6. Laceration, perforation, tear, or puncture of organ or body part occurring during an invasive procedure							
7. Wrong procedure performed or procedure performed on wrong patient							
8. Postoperative complications							
9. Adverse drug reaction							
10. Acute MI or CVA within 48 hours of surgical procedure							
11. Cardiac or respiratory arrest							
12. Neurological deficit not present on admission							
13. Patient physically injured while hospitalized							
14. Hospital-acquired (nosocomial) infection							
15. Hospital-acquired decubitis ulcer							
16. Death							
17. Illegible writing							

Directions   Screeners: when an occurrence is found, date and describe on back.
Secondary/peer reviewers: document any comments/corrective action on back. Complete severity & quality codes on front.
Confirmation of an APO means only that the event did occur & that it is not a routine or expected part of the disease process.

FIGURE 7.TT. Form to document results of the peer review of adverse patient occurrences, including recording of severity code and findings of a second peer reviewer for each occurrence.
SOURCE: *Citro FC, et al: Risky business: The first encounter with APOs.* QRC Advisor 5(2):7, Dec 1988.

Target Diagnosis Patient Care Review Form

Target Diagnosis: __Diabetic Coma or Acidosis_____ ICD-9-CM: __250.0-251.9_____

Patient Identifier: _____Age: _____ Sex: _____

Hospital: _____A-Date: _____ D-Date: _____ TLOS: _____

Primary Care Physician: _____ Specialty: _____

Address: _____ Phone: _____

Criteria: (Obtain information from medical record, physician, or patient)

	Yes	No	N/A
1. The patient is a known diabetic.	——	——	——
2. The patient was on oral hypoglycemics prior to hospitalization.	——	——	——
3. The patient was on insulin prior to hospitalization.	——	——	——
4. Prior to hospitalization, blood sugars were being monitored by the (admission blood sugar _____)	——	——	——
patient.	——	——	——
physician.	——	——	——
5. There were precipitating factors relating to this hospitalization.	——	——	——
If yes, comment.			
6. Prior to hospitalization, a special diet had been prescribed for the patient.	——	——	——
7. There is evidence of patient noncompliance with treatment plan (eg, medications, diet, follow-up visits, etc) within 60 days prior to hospitalization.	——	——	——
If yes, comment.			
8. The patient has received education regarding any area of noncompliance.	——	——	——
9. Condition of fundus (eye) was noted in physical exam.	——	——	——

Reviewer Comments:

Signature: _____ Date: _____

(continued)

Target Diagnosis Patient Care Review Form (continued)

To: Medical Director and/or Designated Peer Reviewer

Date	Comments	Signature

Standard of Care: _____ (+) _____ (+/−) _____ (−) Severity: _____
Date: _____ Signature: _____
_____

TO: QUALITY ASSURANCE COORDINATOR   DATE RECEIVED: _____
Comments:

Referred to Risk Management: _____ No _____ Yes Date of referral: _____

FIGURE 7.UU. Form used in evaluating care received by ambulatory care patients. This reporting form aids in determining whether an inpatient admission indicates a previous problem in quality of care. SOURCE: Solberg LI (HMO Minnesota), Peterson KE (Minnesota Department of Health), Ellis RW (Group Health Plan, IN), Romness K (Share Health Plan): The Minnesota Project: A Focused Approach to Ambulatory Care Quality Assurance, *1987.*

Initial Evaluation Form

Date _____ Department _____ Evaluator _____

Chart Number _____ Age _____ Sex _____ Admit date _____

Admitting Diagnosis _____ Discharge Diagnosis _____

Admitting Physician _____

Important Aspect of Care _____

Indicators (check those not met):

☐ 1. _____

_____

☐ 2. _____

_____

☐ 3. _____

_____

☐ 4. _____

_____

☐ 5. _____

_____

☐ 6. _____

_____

☐ 7. _____

_____

Initial Evaluator Comments:

Recommendation: _____ Further information
_____ Further review
_____ No further review

Disposition: _____

_____

FIGURE 7.VV. Example of form for initial evaluation of cases for which indicator thresholds for evaluation have been reached.

TAKE ACTIONS TO IMPROVE CARE

STEP 8

If the evaluation identifies an opportunity for improvement, staff should decide what action is necessary. A plan of corrective action identifies *who* or *what* is expected to change; *who* is responsible for implementing action; *what* action is appropriate in view of the cause, scope, and severity of the issue; and *when* change is expected to occur. If a needed action exceeds the department director's or QA coordinator's authority, recommendations should be forwarded to the body that can authorize action. A record of actions taken should be maintained.

Some possible actions include

- (for systems problems) changes in communication channels, changes in organizational structures and processes, adjustments in staffing, and changes in equipment or chart forms;

- (for knowledge problems) in-service education, continuing education, making accessible data or scientific reports, and circulating informational material; and

- (for behavior problems) informal or formal counseling, changes in assignments, and disciplinary action.

The most common problem in monitoring and evaluation is failure to take effective actions once an opportunity for improvement or problem has been identified.

Once you've identified an approach to improving care, take action. This is not a step inherently requiring forms; it is an action-oriented step.

Improving care and service is the *raison d'etre* of monitoring and evaluation; this is why it is so important that a health care organization actually take actions to improve care. It is important to keep records of what action staff recommends taking, what action is finally decided upon and approved, who is supposed to take the action and when, and what action is actually taken. Forms to record what actions are taken are also part of Step 10 (discussed beginning on page 211). As in Figure 8.B., a cumulative record of all QA-related actions taken might be kept.

Key Factors for Definitive Assessment and Improvement Action Plan

WHO or WHAT needs to improve or change
Patient ☐
Provider ☐
Organization ☐
Health care environment ☐

WHAT needs to be changed
Knowledge ☐	Policy ☐	Laws ☐
Skills ☐	Procedures ☐	Economy ☐
Attitudes ☐	Facilities/ equipment ☐	

WHICH actions will be taken
Education ☐	Individual ☐
Counseling ☐	Group ☐
Sanctions ☐	Facility ☐
Administrative ☐	Community ☐

HOW will actions be implemented _____
Details of action (education program or policy change) _____
Person(s) responsible for implementing action _____

HOW LONG will implementation phase last _____

HOW MUCH will action cost _____
Personnel time _____ Indirect costs _____
Resources _____

FIGURE 8.A. *Questionnaire to guide the decision on what actions to take to improve care.*
SOURCE: *Adapted from Williamson JW, Ostrow PC, Braswell HR:* Health Accounting for Quality Assurance. *Rockville, MD: American Occupational Therapy Association, 1981, p 64.*

Summary of Actions Taken as a Result of Quality Assurance Chart Reviews*

	Antibiotics	Sentinel Diseases**	Inpatient Admissions	Drug Reactions
Charts reviews (N = 247)	128	66	17	36
Actions taken: None	79	37	13	35
Patient contacted to come in for follow-up	1	2	1	0
Case discussed with practitioner	47	9	2	1
Staff education	0	4	0	0
Staffing change	3	24	9	2
Policy or procedure change	15	3	4	0
Equipment/supplies improvement	4	1	8	9
Other	1	15	2	0

* Based on biweekly chart reviews conducted from January 4, 1988 through January 6, 1989. Charts for all patients for whom any of the topics applied were reviewed.

** **Sentinel diseases**	**Patients**
Chlamydia	31
Cervical dysplasia	20
Gonorrhea	7
Pneumonia	7
Hepatitis	1
Positive rapid plasma reagin (RPR; syphillis)	0

FIGURE 8.B. *Monitoring and evaluation action summary with actions taken over a given period grouped by category, for presentation to the executive committee or governing board.*
SOURCE: *Adapted from Hoskins EJ: A quality assurance program for a state university student health center. QRB 15(10):325, Oct 1989.*

Guide for Action to Improve Care

Department _____ Date _____
Important aspect of care:
Indicator:
Threshold for evaluation:
Results of monitoring:
Probable reasons for variation/deficiency:

Opportunity for improvement identified:

Corrective action suggested/recommended:

Estimated date of completion of corrective action:
Date recommended action reviewed by QA:
Person responsible for action taken:
Other responsible persons and resources identified to help with chosen course(s) of action
(eg, resource people, in-service programs):

Dates each step of action was taken:

Actual date of completion of corrective action:
Did collected data show hope for improvement?
Is further action planned:
Next monitoring period for this indicator:

Figure 8.C. Form to record what action staff recommends taking, what action is finally decided upon and approved, who is to take the action and when, and what action is actually taken.

Ongoing Monitoring Report

_____ Department

_____ Quarter, 19_____

_____ Through _____, 19_____

Title: Evaluation of Skin Integrity_____

I. PURPOSE: 1. Evaluate nurse compliance to Patient Care Standard for the Nursing Diagnosis: "Skin Integrity Impairment."

2. Evaluate patient outcomes.

II. Total number (Process Criteria) reviewed: _____
Total number compliant: _____
Total percent compliant: _____

III. STANDARD/COMPARATIVE DATA (Threshold for evaluation):   The standard is 85%

IV. CRITERIA: *

Process Criteria	This Quarter	Last Quarter	Average/Quarter Last Year
A. Skin integrity assessed @ 8 hours			
B. Interventions documented @ 24 hours			
C. Patient repositioned @ 2–4 hours if immobile			
D. Use of appropriate assistive devices			
E. Mobilization of patient			
F. Daily dressing change			
G. Plan of care documented on patient care plan			
H. Average compliance			
Outcome Criteria			
I. Pressure sore minimized/healed			

V. SUMMARY OF FINDINGS:

VI. RECOMMENDATIONS AND/OR FOLLOW UP:

_____   _____
Department Manager   Date

_____   _____
Administration   Date

_____   _____
Director of Quality Assurance   Date

FIGURE 8.D. _Form for recording monitoring and evaluation findings and recommendations for action._
SOURCE: _Ravenswood Hospital Medical Center, Chicago. Used with permission._

ASSESS ACTIONS AND DOCUMENT IMPROVEMENT

S T E P

9

Staff should next determine whether the action was successful. The findings from continued monitoring (or from special follow-up monitoring, for areas not subject to ongoing monitoring) will provide evidence to determine whether actions are effective. If, for example, the level of performance for the given indicator is unchanged, the action may not have been successful; if the level of performance improves notably, the action was probably successful. Even if care appears to be improved, monitoring is continued to ensure sustained improvement.

The results of continued monitoring and evaluation activities should be documented to provide a record of the efficacy of actions taken. If the quality of care in a specific area does not improve, then the deficiency, its cause, and the action taken to improve it should be assessed. New action should then be taken, and, once again, the effectiveness of the action should be assessed.

Monitoring is continued. Ongoing monitoring should continue for the selected important aspects of care and service. When feedback from outside the ongoing monitoring process triggers evaluation, the leaders should decide the appropriate follow-up monitoring. They may decide that, for example, subsequent patient-satisfaction questionnaires will provide sufficient information. They may also decide that ongoing monitoring needs to be initiated; then, a team would identify indicators, thresholds, and data sources for the aspect of care, which would be added to the ongoing monitoring activities. The important aspects of care that have been chosen for ongoing monitoring and the indicators should be regularly reviewed to determine whether the priorities for ongoing monitoring should be changed or whether the indicators should be revised.

Forms used for Step 9 are highly similar to those used for Step 10 (ie, communicating findings) and are therefore grouped together under Step 10.

STEP 10 COMMUNICATE FINDINGS ORGANIZATIONWIDE

It is essential that monitoring and evaluation information be communicated to the necessary individuals and departments in the organization. Such dissemination helps ensure that QA findings are used to improve care throughout the organization, that activities are not duplicated, and that relevant findings are used in the periodic reappraisal of practitioners (see Appendix B) on using monitoring and evaluation findings in practitioner evaluation). Systematically communicating monitoring and evaluation results helps integrate quality assurance program activities within the organization's managerial structure and contributes to the detection of trends, performance patterns, or potential problems that affect more than one service or group.

The reporting of information can be accomplished by routing summary reports of monitoring and evaluation activities, graphs of findings, or minutes of meetings at which monitoring and evaluation activities are discussed. Once an opportunity for improvement has been identified and action taken, reports and minutes of these QA proceedings should list the *conclusions* of evaluation, *recommendations, actions taken,* and *follow-up* indicating the effectiveness of the action taken.

In reporting monitoring and evaluation activities, some hospitals confuse actions and recommendations. Recommendations are necessary when the person(s) carrying out the evaluation lack the authority to carry out the action they deem necessary to improve quality. Also, conclusions and actions are sometimes confused. Conclusions involve a statement of the root problem, while actions call for a statement of what staff did or are going to do about it.

Monitoring and evaluation activities and results should be reported to the organizationwide QA program, administrative and clinical leaders, governing board, and other appropriate groups and/or individuals (eg, practitioners affected by the QA activities in question). The channels and frequency of communication should be delineated in the health care organization's written QA plan. To provide consistency in reporting methods across departments, the facility's QA plan should specify the method to be used.

The frequency of reporting is determined by the number of data-collection activities conducted. Monthly reports on some activities may be necessary, whereas others may be reported quarterly or semiannually.

Many of the forms included in this compendium as part of the chapters on taking action (Step 8) and, especially, evaluating care (Step 7) would also be suitable for reporting QA findings. A calendar for the scheduling of a department's monitoring and evaluation activity reports could be structured something like the data-collection organization calendars in Figures 6.C. through 6.E.

Figures 10.A. and 10.B. are a questionnaire and table used in planning the reporting of monitoring and evaluation activities.

Variations on forms for reporting findings, conclusions, recommendations, actions, and assessments of the effectiveness of actions comprise Figures 10.C. through 10.J. These tools help staff members follow a monitoring and evaluation episode from problem identification to solution. Figure 10.C. is an example of a quality improvement "storyboard" or "picture book" used to efficiently present process improvement studies to management. (See the chapter on evaluation of care [Step 7] for more ideas on how charts and graphs can also be used to document improvement.)

Figure 10.K. is a report designed to show a particular practitioner his or her own rate of indicator compliance.

Two follow-up forms help keep staff up to date on the changing status of particular aspects of care and service being evaluated (Figures 10.L. and 10.M.). Such forms can be important way to keep track of many evaluations and actions being taken to improve care and service.

Figures 10.N. through 10.Q. are especially appropriate for reporting quality-related data to the governing board. Such reporting should be summarized, but contain enough information for board members to get a good picture of how well the organization is doing.

Monitoring and Evaluation Report Generation/Information Dissemination

What reports are generated?

How are they generated (manual versus computer)?

Who creates/sends reports?

Who receives reports?

How often is each type of report circulated?

What levels of reporting exist?

   Intradepartmental:

   Interdepartmental:

     Horizontal:

     Vertical (reporting chain):

What reporting formats are used for different types of staff members?

What kind of reports are used to report monitoring and evaluation findings to patient care staff (eg, physicians, nurses, technicians)?

What kind of summary reports are presented to the governing board?

Are reporting formats easy to understand?

Have staff complained about reporting formats?

Are reports unnecessarily negative in tone?

Do reporting mechanisms maintain staff and patient confidentiality as much as possible?

Is there reason to believe that administration and patient care staff actually read monitoring and evaluation reports? If not, why not?

What do different levels of staff want to see on monitoring and evaluation reports?

Is the information on reports objective and scientific in tone?

Does reporting help reduce duplication of activities and contribute to the detection of trends that affect more than one service or group?

Figure 10.A. Questionnaire used in evaluating reports of monitoring and evaluation information.

QA Reporting Mechanism Procedure

COMPONENT OF REPORTING MECHANISM	PROCEDURE	RESPONSIBILITY
1. Preapproved QA indicators/outcomes • general (hospitalwide) • unit-specific (departmental)	Post on unit for purpose of ongoing monitoring	All personnel
2. Identification of occurrence or problem	Step 1 - QA Notice QA coordinator notified by phone, beeper or in writing depending on severity of occurrence and/or outcome.	All personnel
3. Response/Intervention	Immediate response and intervention to high priority occurrences. Otherwise, QA notices placed in a designated area on the unit and picked up on rounds once each shift by QA.	Person reporting occurrence QA Coordinator Administrator Physician Any appropriate department
4. Evaluation	Step 2 - QA Report and/or Risk Identification Report (RIR) QA Coordinator will forward report to unit for completion. Completed QA report goes to Department Director.	Person reporting occurrence Department Director Any appropriate department
Monthly Summary Report Quality Assurance Unit (QAU) • conclusions • recommendations • action taken • monitoring	Summary of QAU activity compiled and reported to QA Coordinator by the 5th day of the following month to include: 1) indicators with analysis of casual factors 2) focus review reports reflecting the QA Schedule prepared by each QAU according to the QA Plan <u>Reporting format</u> <u>Denominator</u> = total number of cases, procedures, etc, performed <u>Numerator</u> = number of occurrences that "fell out" <u>Index</u> by % = Numerator ÷ Denominator = % <u>Analysis/Trending</u> = Why each occurrence happened and, if preventable, how. Problems resolvable at QAU level -complete cause, action, follow-up in report to QA Coordinator QA Coordinator collects departmental monthly summaries; compiles data to present to Medical Staff QA Committee	Department Director or Department QA Designee
6. Quarterly Trend Analysis	Problems identified in quarterly trend analysis of QA indicators focus review or other methods Problems which cannot be resolved after three months at the QAU level and are referred to Medical Staff QA Committee	Department Directors/Medical Directors QA Coordinator with input from Department Director/Medical Director
7. Annual Evaluation	Review and evaluate for effectiveness	Department Director QA Coordinator Medical Staff QA Committee Administration

FIGURE 10.B. *Matrix shows procedure and persons responsible for various aspects of monitoring and evaluation reporting.*
SOURCE: *Laura A. Crotti Rosio. Used with permission.*

Quality Improvement Storyboard

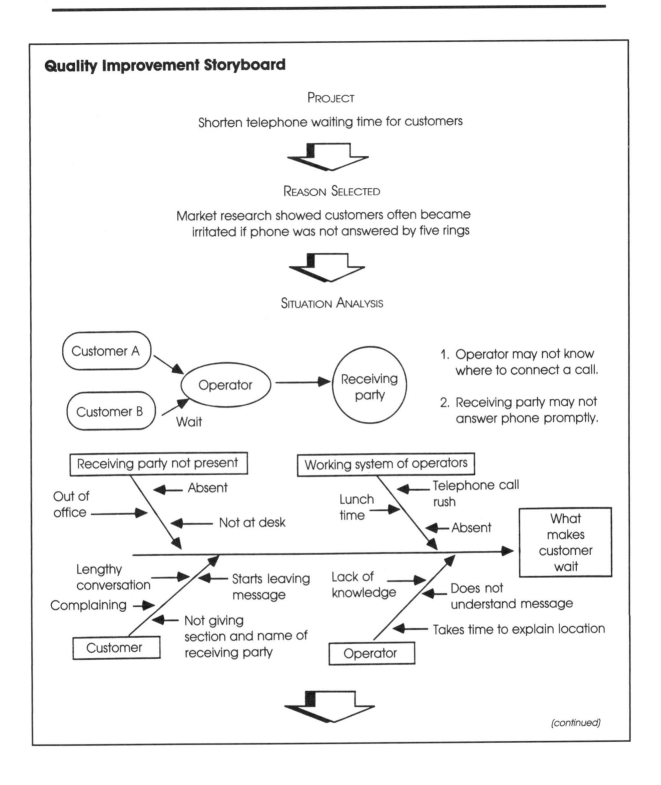

PROJECT

Shorten telephone waiting time for customers

REASON SELECTED

Market research showed customers often became
irritated if phone was not answered by five rings

SITUATION ANALYSIS

Customer A

Customer B

Operator

Wait

Receiving
party

1. Operator may not know
   where to connect a call.

2. Receiving party may not
   answer phone promptly.

Receiving party not present

Absent

Out of
office

Not at desk

Working system of operators

Telephone call
rush

Lunch
time

Absent

What
makes
customer
wait

Lengthy
conversation

Complaining

Starts leaving
message

Not giving
section and name of
receiving party

Customer

Lack of
knowledge

Does not
understand message

Takes time to explain location

Operator

(continued)

Quality Improvement Storyboard (continued)

DATA COLLECTION

Check Sheet

Reason / Date	No one present in the section receiving the call	Receiving party not present	Only one operator		Total
June 4	\\\\	⫴⫴ \	⫴⫴ ⫴⫴ \		24
June 5	⫴⫴	⫴⫴ \\\	⫴⫴ ⫴⫴ \\\\		32
June 6	⫴⫴ \	\\\	⫴⫴ ⫴⫴ \		28
⋮	⋮	⋮	⋮		
June 15	⫴⫴	⫴⫴	⫴⫴ \\\		25

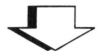

DATA ANALYSIS

Reasons why callers had to wait

		Daily average	Total number
A	One operator (partner out of the office)	14.3	172
B	Receiving party not present	6.1	73
C	No one present in the section receiving the call	5.1	61
D	Section and name of receiving party not given	1.6	19
E	Inquiry about branch office locations	1.3	16
F	Other reasons	0.8	10
	Total	29.2*	351

*6% of calls had long waits

(continued)

Quality Improvement Storyboard (continued)

PARETO DIAGRAM

A	One operator (partner out of the office)
B	Receiving party not present
C	No one present in the section receiving the call
D	Section and name of receiving party not given
E	Inquiry about branch office locations
F	Other reasons

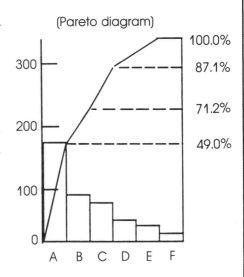

(Pareto diagram)

GOAL

Reduce calls with long waits to zero

ACTIONS

1. Helper operator brought in from clerical section to substitute while each of two regular operators went to lunch.

2. Asked all employees to leave messages when leaving their desks.

3. Compiled directory listing personnel and their respective jobs.

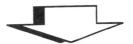

(continued)

Quality Improvement Storyboard (continued)

EVALUATION

Comparisons of before and after

	Reasons why callers had to wait	Total number Before	Total number After	Daily average Before	Daily average After
A	One operator (partner out of the office)	172	15	14.3	1.2
B	Receiving party not present	73	17	6.1	1.4
C	No one present in the section receiving the call	61	20	5.1	1.7
D	Section and name of receiving party not given	19	4	1.6	0.3
E	Inquiry about branch office locations	16	3	1.3	0.2
F	Other reasons	10	0	0.8	0
		351	59	29.2*	4.8

*6% of calls had long waits

Period: 12 days from Aug. 17 to 30

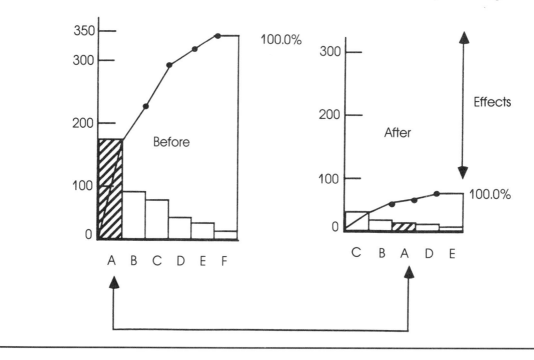

FIGURE 10.C. A quality improvement "storyboard" or "picture book" can be developed to show management and staff what steps were taken to evaluate an aspect of care or service (in this case, telephone waiting times) and improve it. (Figure 7.W. is also a type of quality improvement storyboard.) Consistent with a continuous quality improvement approach, the storyboard displays the milestones of a quality improvement team's efforts through a series of flowchart-like entries, including graphs and descriptive pictures. The boxes lead the reader through the project's main findings, conclusions, and actions in a simple, understandable fashion. The project team leader and/or quality advisor should fill in the first two or three entries prior to the team's first meeting.
SOURCE: This example of a Picture Book format is adapted from a classic anecdote from the brochure The Quest for Higher Quality: The Deming Prize and Quality Control, RICOH of America, Inc. It appears in The Team Handbook © 1988 Joiner Associates, Inc, and is reproduced by the Joint Commission with permission.

Monitoring and Evaluation Tracking Log

Department: _____ Responsible Individual: _____

Indicator	Problem Description	Date Identified	Problem Analysis (Step 7)	Corrective Action (Step 8)	Follow-up Action if problem persists (Step 9)	Results of Actions	Date Resolved	Evidence of Resolution

FIGURE 10.D. Log for tracking monitoring and evaluation activities.

Quality Assessment Summary/Monitor				
MONTH	ASPECT OF CARE EVALUATED	EVALUATION CONCLUSIONS	ACTION	EVIDENCE OF RESOLUTION
Jan				
Feb				
Mar				
Apr				
May				
Jun				
Jul				
Aug				
Sep				
Oct				
Nov				
Dec				

FIGURE 10.E. Tracking of evaluations and actions to improve care displayed month by month.

Unplanned Admissions to ICU Department: Family Practice

Date: Jan.–Mar., 1989

Phys. #	Case #	Patient Profile	Reviewed by	Action to date	Action Required	Outcome
103036	1	47-yr-old diabetic admitted to 23 Hr Outpatient Unit. History of fever and headache, increased WBC and antibiotic therapy for 2 wks. 3 visits to ER. Admitted with meningitis and expired.	ER, family practice, risk management			QA liaison reviewed. Letter of response to file.
103034	2	86-yr-old presented in ER with tarry stools and tachycardia. History of peptic ulcer. Patient admitted to telemetry without assessment for GI bleed. Had massive hemorrhage with hemoglobin to 5.3.	ER, family practice			Family practice QA liaison reviewed with physician. To file.
103053	3	24-yr-old with history of syncope admitted via ER to telemetry. Had 7-sec. pause-junctional rhythm. Required temporary pacemaker.	Nursing QA			Nurse/Nurse Manager recognized error, counseling on protocol followed.

FIGURE 10.F. Reporting form on actions taken to address a sentinel event (unplanned admission to the intensive care unit) involving individual practitioners.
SOURCE: Adapted from Memorial Hospital, Hollywood, FL. Used with permission.

Drug Usage Evaluation Status Report

Topic: Education of Asthma Cases

DATE & SOURCE	SPECIFIC PROBLEM	CAUSE AND ATTRIBUTION	ACTION WHAT/WHEN	RESP. PARTY
6/87 Nursing QM Committee	Evidence that patients not fully informed of all relevant self-care activities; simultaneous (and probably related) problem concerning patient compliance with self-care regimen.	Patient information check list has yet to be fully implemented; presently no systematic way of ensuring all relevant instructions passed along to patients, which may result in problems with patient compliance. In addition, problems with follow-up appointment reminder system might be affecting that particular aspect of patient compliance.	Beginning 7/87, the first visits of all new asthma cases will be monitored to ensure that records contain evience of necessary self-care instruction; monitor will continue for 4 months. After completion of the above monitor a review of the follow-up appointment reminder system will be considered.	Dept of Nsg. Nsg. QM Comm.

NEXT REVIEW DATE	STATUS AND FURTHER ACTION	NEXT REVIEW DATE	STATUS AND FURTHER ACTION	NEXT REVIEW DATE	STATUS AND FURTHER ACTION	SOLVED
8/87	Fifteen asthma cases were monitored. Of these, almost half (47%) did not contain the information check list. Of the 8 cases containing the check list, half were missing at least one item of information. Reminder memoranda were sent to all nurses reiterating the new check list policy and reemphasizing its importance vis-a-vis the rate of recidivism for asthma patients.	9/87	Eighteen cases were monitored. Fourteen (78%) of the records reviewed contained the information check list. At least one item of information was missing in 10 (71%) of these cases. Nurses who continue to disregard directive to complete check list were required to attend meeting held by DON, who personally stressed the need to complete the check list.	10/87	Fourteen cases were monitored. Information check lists were completed in each case, and only 2 (14%) were missing at least one item of information. The Nursing QM committee concluded that the information check list procedure for asthma cases was now fully implemented, and began considering other monitors to ensure patient compliance.	10/87

Figure 10.G. Form facilitates tracking of a particular problem through successive actions to improve care.

Source: *Joseph ED, Brown R, Celestin C:* Protocols for Evaluating Ambulatory Care, Volume 2: Drug Usage Evaluation. *Chicago: Care Communications, 1988, pp 150-151.*

Management Referral Report Form

Part I   Issue/Concern (To be completed by referring department/committee)
(Attach additional paperwork if necessary)

Refer to:

_____
Individual/department/committee

_____   _____
Individual completing report   Department/committee chairperson

Part II   Review (To be completed by referring department/committee)
(Attach additional paperwork if necessary)

Findings:

Conclusions:

Recommendations:

Actions:

_____   _____
Individual completing report   Department/committee chairperson

Part III   QA Review (To be completed by QA)

Review: Present at:

Actions taken: QM Committee _____

                                                   MSEC _____
Feedback to department/committee
                                                   Refer to:

_____   _____
QM   QM Physician Advisor

Part IV   Feedback (To be completed by referring department)

Review of actions taken

Issue resolved _____   ☐ No further action necessary

Issue not resolved _____

Refer to: _____

_____

Signature

Figure 10.H. Form that allows both a clinical department and the QA department to review monitoring and evaluation findings, conclusions, recommendations and actions taken.
Source: Longo DR, Ciccone KR, Lord JT: Integrated Quality Assessment: A Model for Concurrent Review. *Chicago: American Hospital Publishing, Inc, 1989, p 158.*

Impact Assessment

Results of study identified needs in one or more of the following areas
  (Please circle applicable areas):

knowledge	procedure _____
resource	supervision _____
performance	documentation _____
policy	communication _____
motivation	other (please specify): _____

Effect of corrective action:

_____ Corrective action has been effective in preventing or minimizing problems. No further evaluation is necessary.

_____ The situation has improved but continued monitoring is necessary.

_____ The situation has not improved significantly. Further action is required. (Specify plan of action): _____

_____

_____

Impact on practice, policy, or procedure: (Indicate ALL departments/services affected):

_____

_____

_____

_____

Signs of real improvement:

Patient Care:

_____

_____

_____

_____

Staff:

_____

_____

_____

_____

Organization:

_____

_____

_____

_____

Figure 10.I. *Form that offers a more subjective approach to identifying a need for improvement and recording whether corrective action was effective.*
Source: *Adapted from UCLA Medical Center, Los Angeles. Used with permission.*

Monitoring and Evaluation Tracking and Reporting Form

Department _____ Date _____

Important aspect of care:

Indicator:

Threshold for evaluation:

Data findings:

Was an opportunity for evaluation identified? Yes _____ No _____

Conclusions of data evaluation, including specific opportunity for improvement identified and cause of variation in patient care:

Recommendations (if a needed action exceeded the authority of the department):

Actions taken (include dates):

Person(s) responsible for action taken:

Follow-up action taken, if any (include dates):

Improvement documented:

Is further action planned?

Date problem resolved:

Evidence of resolution:

Most recent data level for this indicator:

Next date that data collected for this indicator will be compared to the threshold for evaluation:

Routing of this report:

FIGURE 10.J. *Forms for tracking the monitoring and evaluation process from problem identification to solution.*

Health Maintenance Summary Report

Physician's name:
Date of report: 9/30/89

This report summarizes your preventive health care during the period 7/1/89 through 9/30/89. During this period you saw 94 patients. A total of 1325 patients were seen by all physicians in the medical clinic.

The completion rate (expressed as a percentage) was calculated according to the following equation:

$$\text{Completion rate} = (\text{number completed}/\text{number indicated}) \times 100$$

The number completed and the number indicated does not include patients who were offered the preventive health care intervention but refused. A completed preventive health care intervention appears on the doctor's order sheet under the heading "completed" while an indicated intervention appears under the heading "indicated." An indicated intervention is dependent upon the person's age, sex, diagnoses, and when (if ever) the intervention was last performed.

	PERCENT COMPLETED	
INTERVENTION	YOUR SCORE	CLINIC SCORE
Pap smear	42	60
Breast exam	68	58
Mammography	35	55
Hemoccult × 3	86	61
Rectal exam	75	63
Sigmoidoscopy	90	62
Influenza vaccine	82	90
Pneumonia vaccine	100	88
Tetanus vaccine	45	57
Cholesterol	72	61
Urinalysis	55	72
Ophthalmology exam	65	70
D.M. diet consult	25	41
Glycohemoglobin	12	48
Urine microalbumin	18	32
Electrocardiogram	78	81
Electrolytes/Bun	83	74

FIGURE 10.K. *Report to a particular practitioner on his or her own monitoring scores compared to a clinic's overall performance.*
SOURCE: *York Hospital Medical Clinic, York, PA. Used with permission.*

Evaluation/Problem Tracking Summary

Aspect of Care/ Problem	JULY	AUG	SEPT	OCT	NOV	DEC	JAN	FEB	MAR	APR	MAY	JUNE

KEY: PI = PROBLEM IDENTIFIED
FU = FOLLOW-UP
PR = PROBLEM RESOLVED
SR = SUSTAINED RESOLUTION (AT 6 MONTHS)   UNIT: _____

FIGURE 10.L. *Problem tracking summary. Form helps keep staff up to date on the changing status of particular aspects of care and service being evaluated and improved.*
SOURCE: Jayne Resek, associate director, Quality Healthcare Resources, Inc, a not-for-profit subsidiary of the Joint Commission, Oakbrook Terrace, IL.

QA Activity/Problem Status Log Index

Department: _____

QA Chairperson: _____

| Unit | Activity/ Problem | FILE # | IMPLEMENTATION DATES | | | | STATUS OF ACTION PLAN | | | | | STATUS OF ACTIVITY/PROBLEM | | | Comments |
			Log	Action Plan	Study/ Pilot	Plan Review	Pending Review	Pending Policy	Pending Approval	Follow-up	On-going	Follow-up	On-going	Resolved	

FIGURE 10.M. *Matrix helps track the status of action plans.*
SOURCE: *Hospital of the University of Pennsylvania, Philadelphia. Used with permission.*

Quarterly Quality Assurance Report to the Governing Board

	Current period	Year-to-date	Comments

QUALITY ASSURANCE
Mortality rate
- Medicare patients _____
- All other patients _____

Infection rate _____

Medical staff reviews
- Number of cases reviewed
  per 100 patient discharges _____
- % meeting
  standard of care _____

Clinical service departments
- Number of problem
  areas identified _____
- Number of problem
  issues resolved _____

PRO-identified events
- Level 1 and 2 (minor) _____
- Level 3 and 4 (major) _____

UTILIZATION REVIEW
Nonreimbursed days
- Medicare _____
- Medicaid _____
- Other third-party payer _____
- Days of unnecessary
  hospitalization attributed
  to discharge delays _____

RISK MANAGEMENT
Professional liability—litigated claims
- Number opened _____
- Number closed _____
- Number pending _____

Professional liability—nonlitigated claims
- Number opened _____
- Number closed _____
- Number pending _____

Workers' compensation loss ratio _____

PATIENT SATISFACTION
Composite survey scores
- Overall _____
- Inpatient _____
- Outpatient _____

Reported patient complaints _____

FIGURE 10.N. *Format for a quarterly report to the governing board, including reporting on utilization review and risk management and patient satisfaction.*
SOURCE: *Spath P: Hospitals must take proactive role in defining high-quality health care.* Hospital Peer Review *13(1), Jan 1988.*

Patient Care Provider Competence Assessment

HOSPITAL _____

DATE   _____

This report reflects review of the competence of direct care providers for the period _____ through
_____.

The following types of employees provide patient care and are not subject to the medical staff privilege
delineation process. For these provider groups competence is shown by a satisfactory annual evaluation.

CATEGORY	NUMBER OF EMPLOYEES	NUMBER WITH SATISFACTORY EVALUATIONS	NUMBER RECEIVING MARGINAL EVALUATION AND ACTION			NUMBER OF OVERDUE EVALUATIONS
			NUMBER ON PROBATION	NUMBER RESIGNED OR TERMINATED	OTHER (PLEASE SPECIFY)	
Nurses						
Dietitians						
EKG Technicians						
Emergency Medical Technicians						
Laboratory Assistants						
Laboratory Technologists						
Nurse's Aides						
Occupational Therapist						
Speech Pathologists						
Surgical Technicians						
Other _____						
Other _____						
Other _____						
Totals						

Complied by _____ Approved by _____

FIGURE 10.O. Tool to help assess the competence of personnel providing direct patient care. The categories of employees cited are not exhaustive (or as complete as may be necessary.) This report may be used to summarize the results of the performance assessment process for governing board members.

Performance • Evaluation Summary

DEPARTMENT OF <u>MEDICINE</u>   DATE <u>MARCH 1990</u>

SUBMITTED BY <u>WILLIAM SMITH, MD, CHAIRMAN</u>

	JANUARY			FEBRUARY			MARCH		
	No. Cases Abstracted	No. Cases Questioned	No. 3,4,5	No Cases Abstracted	No. Cases Questioned	No. 3,4,5	No. Cases Abstracted	No. Cases Questioned	No. 3,4,5
Blood Use	32	3	1	26	4	2	29	7	3
Drugs/Antibiotics	96	52	8	82	39	9	87	47	6
MR/DRG/UM	111	100	90	94	80	60	50	40	40
Surgical Case Review	N/A ----			-------------			-------------		--------------
Special Care Units	39	7	0	27	4	1	31	5	1
Mortality (Deaths)	3	3	0	2	2	1	4	4	0

COMMENTS

(1) There were no "5's" (cases which might require Board action) in March.

(2) The 3 blood use cases judged "3's" and "4's" in March were instances of use of whole blood rather than specific components . . . an unacceptable practice because of increased risk to the patient, and inefficient use of blood and blood products . . . by three different physicians, who have been counselled.

(3) The continuing high number of "3's" and "4's" in MR/DRG/UM (Medical Records, Diagnosis-Related Group financial data and Utilization Management) reflects continued lack of attention to legible, informational and timely completion of patients' medical records.

(4) The four deaths were all anticipated on admission. Patients presented with either terminal stages of chronic disease, or untreatable acute conditions.

(5) The one "4" in Special Care Unit case review is the same issue, in the practice of the same staff member, as the one "4" noted in February. No Board action is requested at this time.

FIGURE 10.P. Format for reporting summarized results of quality evaluations or peer review to the governing body. Those questioned cases where more serious problems were noted are given scores of 3, 4, or 5 (the latter being the most negative score). A brief narrative section fleshes out and explains the implications of numerical scores.
SOURCE: *Thompson RE: The Governing Body Member's and CEO's Guide to Medical Staff Organization and Responsibilities. Dunedin, FL: Thompson, Mohr & Associates, Inc, 1989, pp 101, 103.*

Report to the Board on "Occurrence Screening System"

Report To: *Board QA Committee*   **Hospital:** *Anywhere General*

Month: *August*   **Year:** *1981*

No. Hospital Admissions: 203   **No. Records Screened:** *203*   **No. APOs** *32*

No. ER Visits: *948*   **No. Records Screened:** *948*   **No. APOs** *46*

No. Incident Reports: *32*   **No. Potential Claims:** *1*   **No. Actual Claims:** *None*

No. Nosocomial Infections: *3*   **No. Deaths:** *None*

Trends/Occurrences	Action(s)	Follow-Up
Medical Staff — Trends **Medical Records** 1. 15% of surgeries had no op report dicated 4-6 weeks after discharge. If no improvement, suspension policy to be included in rules and regulations. 2. Records with consent problems a) 10 - no informed consent b) 8 - no date or time c) 1 - incomplete 3. One physician consistently refuses to complete medical records on time.	1. Memos sent to involved surgeons reminding them of 24-hour policy and that it will be enforced. 2. Copy recent edition of CHA consent manual and send to entire staff; invite claims representative to speak on this issue at next staff meeting. 3. Physician put on notice of suspension until records completed.	1. Medical records to report weekly to Chief of Surgery on late op reports. 2. Good discussion at meeting 9/16/81; physicians agreed to make informed consent note part of preop check list. Continuous monitoring for consents is in progress and shows improvement. 3. Records completed; continuous monitor with monthly report to QA Committee.
Complications 1. Three patients had breakdown of episiotomy within 2 days (different physicians). 2. Three patients on anticoagulants admitted for bleeding problems (one physician).	1. Immediate investigation identified defective suture lot; suture removed. 2. Control and monitoring of anticoagulants discussed with physician by Chief of Medicine.	1. No further problem. 2. Continuous monitoring; no further problem.
Utilization 1. Two physicians consistently write illegible notes so reason for increased LOS cannot be determined.	1. Physicians notified of progress.	1. Continuous monitoring of problem. To be called each time entry is illegible.

(continued)

Report to the Board on "Occurrence Screening System" (continued)

TRENDS/OCCURRENCES	ACTION(S)	FOLLOW-UP
Medical Staff Occurrences **Complications** 1. Patient had chest pain postop cholecystectomy; ECG done but not read and patient discharged; returned DOA with myocardial infarction.	1. Ad Hoc Committee convened to review case; reported to claims; discussed with surgeon. New policies on reading ECGs on weekends and medical consultation on surgical patients written.	1. No claims activity to date. Administration asked to support ECG telecommunication program.
Utilization 1. Inappropriate admission of a severe burn — patient not isolated; transferred 24 hours later	1. Rewrite policies on admission and isolation of burn patients; ask burn center to write critique of pretransfer care of this patient.	1. Burn Center wrote critique and sent specialist to discuss burn care at last medical staff meeting. Patient did well after transfer.
Antibiotics 1. Inappropriate use of Keflin in patient with renal stones.	1. Memo to physician; set up concurrent screening criteria for cephalosporins.	1. Concurrent monitoring shows continued problem. QA Committee will follow-up and report back.
Medical Records 1. Physician destroyed 2 days of progress notes and rewrote them.	1. Physician counselled re: dire legal consequences of altering records.	1. Observation for further problems.
Nursing — Trends 1. Increased numbers of IV infiltrates and skin problems. 2. Intakes and outputs not recorded or totalled accurately. 3. Increased number of infections post-foley catheter insertion.	1. Focused study done on causes of increased infiltrates. 2. Inservice education; calculators put on each unit. 3. All shifts to have inservice in Sept.	1. Infiltrates decreased over past month since micron filters being used on all IVs. 2. Improvement noted in the first month. Continued monitoring. 3. Continued monitoring.
Respiratory Therapy — Trends 1. MA-1 respirators breaking down; discovered that engineer not trained to service these respirators.	1. Engineer sent to take course on servicing MA-1 respirators.	1. To be reevaluated.

FIGURE 10.Q. Two-page format to summarize and report findings of monitoring and evaluation to the governing body. The report gives total numbers of admissions and emergency care visits, number of records screened, and number of adverse patient occurrences noted. The second part of the form summarizes trends/occurrences noted, actions taken to improve care, and follow-up to these actions. **SOURCE:** *Bader & Associates, Inc:* Keys to Better Hospital Governance Through Better Information. *Harrisburg, PA: Hospital Trustee Association of Pennsylvania, 1985, pp 65-66.*

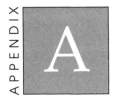

FORMS FOR ANNUAL APPRAISAL OF THE ORGANIZATIONWIDE QA PROGRAM

The objectives, scope, organization, and effectiveness of the health care organization's quality assurance program should be evaluated at least annually and revised as necessary. The program appraisal includes

- evaluating the monitoring and evaluation process to determine its effectiveness;

- comparing the written QA plan with the QA activities that were performed;

- determining whether QA information was communicated accurately and to the appropriate persons or committees; and

- determining whether opportunities for improvement were actively taken and patient care improved.

The annual appraisal of the quality assurance program is intended to evaluate both the effectiveness of the program's components and the program's overall performance. The program should be appraised by an appropriate individual or group (eg, the QA coordinator, the hospital administrator, or a committee appointed by one of those individuals). A comprehensive report should be made to the governing body and group responsible for QA oversight (eg, the QA committee), and shared with professional staff and administration.

There is a plethora of possible methods to annually evaluate the QA program. Although not mandatory, forms can be helpful in guiding the process. Forms for evaluating the QA program are shown as Figures A.1. through A.6. Figure A.7. helps staff evaluate whether they are monitoring the most important aspects of care, whether indicators and peer review are meaningful, and whether monitoring and evaluation is leading to real improvements. Figures A.8. and A.9. are forms to help evaluate the nursing QA program.

Figures A.10. and A.11. get at one of the most important issues: the improvements brought by quality assurance. A big part of evaluating the QA program is simply profiling the improvements in care achieved through monitoring and evaluation and other QA mechanisms.

"Evaluating the QA program involves showing the improvements made through QA and then asking 'How can we improve it?'" says Jean Carroll, the Joint Commission's acting director of standards development.*

Other forms include a questionnaire for collecting data on the satisfaction of clinical staff members with the services and consultations they receive from the organization's QA department (Figure A.12.), and more general survey instruments to measure satisfaction of various segments of the staff with the QA program (Figures A.13. through A.15.).

REFERENCE

* Personal communication between the author and J Carroll, Nov 1990.

Self-Appraisal of Your Quality Assurance Program

DEPARTMENT _____

    Please respond to the following questions and return this form to the Quality Assurance Coordinator. If you have any questions about the information below, please call him/her.

I. An ongoing planned and systematic monitoring and evaluation process of the **quality and appropriateness** of patient care services is implemented.

    a. Define the scope of services provided by your department. The scope of service includes all the major clinical functions for inpatients and outpatients. (eg, evaluation and assessment of patients' needs, Development of treatment plans). See attached for further definition.

        _____
        _____
        _____
        _____

    b. For the scope of service, the important aspects of care in the major clinical functions are identified (ie, Activities that are high-volume, high-risk or problem prone). Please list these below:

        _____
        _____
        _____

    c. List the indicators you monitored over the past 12 months with the time frames for how often the data was evaluated. Use a separate piece of paper if necessary.

    Indicator   Time Frame

        _____
        _____
        _____
        _____

    d. Did you monitor the important aspects of care provided by your department? (Do your Indicators correspond to the items you listed in section b.?)
        _____ Yes   _____ No

    e. Did you use objective, measurable indicators criteria that reflect current knowledge and clinical experience when assessing your quality assurance information? (Did you have threshold for evaluation set-up for each indicator, if needed?)
        _____ Yes   _____ No

(continued)

Self-Appraisal of Your Quality Assurance Program (continued)

    f. Did you evaluate your Indicators according to your specified time frames? (Compare data collected to pre-established criteria)

        _____ Yes   _____ No

      If not, why?

    g. Did you analyze the data further when indicators were not met?

        _____ Yes   _____ No

    h. Did you draw conclusions at each evaluation period?

        _____ Yes   _____ No

    i. Did you revise your indicators when data consistently met standards?

        _____ Yes   _____ No

II. The quality of patient care is improved and identified problems are resolved through actions taken, as appropriate. (Use separate sheets of paper to answer the questions below, if necessary.)

    a. Were problems identified through your monitoring or other QA activities over the past 12 months? List these problems or opportunities for improvement.

       _____

       _____

       _____

       _____

       _____

    b. What action was taken in relation to the problems identified?

       _____

       _____

       _____

       _____

       _____

    c. Were problems followed up and monitored to determine if they were resolved or reduced to an acceptable level?

        _____ Yes   _____ No

    d. What problems did not get resolved? Why?

       _____

       _____

       _____

       _____

    e. Did you document conclusions, problems identified, action taken and follow-up monitoring results?

        _____ Yes   _____ No

    f. Did you report the results of your monitoring activities at your appropriate department/ committee meeting? (Do you share results with members of your department?)

        _____ Yes   _____ No

Medical Staff Departments Only

    f. 1. Did you participate in the design and implementation of monitoring activities?

        _____ Yes   _____ No

      2. How often did your department meet this past year? _____

      3. Was quality assurance the major agenda item at your monthly meetings?

        _____ Yes   _____ No

      4. Did you report the findings of Medical Staff Committee Quality Assurance Activities to your department? (as provided by Quality Assurance Coordinator)

        _____ Yes   _____ No

(continued)

Self-Appraisal of Your Quality Assurance Program (continued)

   5. Do the minutes of your monthly meetings reflect active discussion by department members regarding quality assurance items?

   _____ Yes   _____ No

   6. Do the minutes reflect that conclusions and recommendations are drawn and action taken when problems are identified?

   _____ Yes   _____ No

   7. Are issues which require follow-up reported back to the department and documented in the minutes?

   _____ Yes   _____ No

   8. Were Quality Assurance results used as a parameter for physician reappointment?

   _____ Yes   _____ No

III.   The main goal of quality assurance is improvement in patient care.

   a. What improvements in patient care have resulted directly from the activities of your quality assurance program in the past 12 months?

   b. Did you use the findings of quality assurance activities to evaluate staff performance, modify policies and procedures, change systems, and so on? Please list these.

   c. Were your educational programs, at least in part, based on the findings from monitoring and evaluation activities? Please correlate QA findings with educational programs given by your department.

   d. Please review your present indicators and criteria to determine their clinical importance, effectiveness in identifying problems and improving patient care.

	Yes	No
1. This past year, no problems or opportunities for improvement were identified.		
2. The problems identified impact patient care.		
3. Indicators were based on high volume, high risk, problem prone areas.		

   e. Please list your 1988 Indicators with their corresponding major clinical functions.

   Indicator   Clinical Function

   _____

   _____

   _____

   _____

   _____

   _____

   Completed by: _____

   Administrative Review Signature: _____ Date: _____

FIGURE A.1. *Form used in the annual evaluation of a hospital's QA program.*
SOURCE: *Gail Bronswick, manager, professional services, Quality Healthcare Resources, Inc, a not-for-profit subsidiary of the Joint Commission, Oakbrook Terrace, IL.*

1987 Appraisal Evaluation Scoring Sheet

Department: _____

> 1 = Substantial compliance - consistently meets all major provision of the standard
> 2 = Significant compliance - meets most provisions of the standard
> 3 = Partial compliance   - meets some provisions of the standard
> 4 = Minimal compliance   - meets few provisions of the standard
> 5 = Noncompliance   - fails to meet the provisions of the standard
>
> The necessary revisions/additions will be discussed with each Department that has a deficiency.

SCORE

The department has a planned and systematic process for the monitoring and evaluation of the Quality & Appropriateness of patient care services

	SCORE
- the scope of services are defined	1 2 3 4 5
- the major clinical functions are defined	1 2 3 4 5
- the important aspects of care in the major clinical functions are identified (hi-volume, hi-risk)	1 2 3 4 5

Routine collection of information about the department's services is performed

-Indicators relating to the Q & A of important aspects of care are identified	1 2 3 4 5
- the Department agrees on objective criteria that reflect current knowledge and clinical experience	1 2 3 4 5
- the criteria are used by the department in monitoring and evaluating patient care	1 2 3 4 5
- Data is routinely collected according to specified time frames	1 2 3 4 5
- Periodic assessment of the collected information is performed and measured against the preestablished criteria	1 2 3 4 5

Problems or opportunities to improve care are identified	1 2 3 4 5
- Action is taken as appropriate	1 2 3 4 5
- the effectiveness of the action taken is evaluated	1 2 3 4 5

The findings, conclusions, recommendations, action taken and results of action taken are documented	1 2 3 4 5
- reported through the channels established by the Hospital	1 2 3 4 5
- necessary information is communicated among departments when problems involve more than one department	1 2 3 4 5
- there is evidence of the Director's responsibility for and involvement in the QA activities	1 2 3 4 5
- the results of QA are used in continuing education of department members	1 2 3 4 5
- QA results are used to appraise the competence of those individuals within the department	1 2 3 4 5

(continued)

1987 Appraisal Evaluation Scoring Sheet (continued)

1987 Quality Assurance Program Evaluation
Support Services

Projected Ratings

	Standard #	Characteristic	1	2	3	4	5
	QA 2	The scope of services is defined	2	4			
	QA 3.1	The major clinical functions are defined	13				
*	QA 3.1	The important aspects of care in the major clinical functions are identified (hi-volume, hi-risk)	6	4	2		1
		Routine collection of information about the department's services is collected					
*	QA 3.1	Indicators relating to the Q & A of important aspects of care are identifed	7	5	1		
	QA 3.2	The department agrees on objective criteria that reflect current knowledge and clinical experience	13				
	QA 3.2.1.3	The criteria are used by the department in monitoring and evaluating patient care	13				
	QA 3.1.1	Data is routinely collected according to specified time frames	10	2			
*	QA 3.2.1.2	Periodic assessment of the collected information is performed and measured against the pre-established criteria	10		3		
*	QA 3.3	Problems or opportunities to improve care are identified	9	3			1
*		Action is taken as appropriate	9	3			1
*	QA 4.3	The effectiveness of the action taken is evaluated	11	1			1
	QA 3.4	The findings, conclusions, recommendations, action taken and results of action taken are documented	12	1			
*		Reported through the channels established by the Hospital	9	3			1
	QA 4.2	Necessary information is communicated among departments when problems involve more than one dept.	12	1			
*		There is evidence of the Director's responsibility for and involvement in the QA activities	12				1
*		The results of QA are used in continuing education of department members	7	4			2
	QA 2.5	QA results are used to appraise the competence of those individuals within the department	7	1	2		3
*		New indicators have been developed for 1988 if few problems were identified in 1987	9	2	1		1

(continued)

1987 Appraisal Evaluation Scoring Sheet (continued)

ITEMS RECEIVING A SCORE OF 3, 4, OR 5
EXPLANATION OF RESULTS

Characteristic	Total scores of 3, 4, and 5, and Explanation
The important aspects of care in the major clinical functions are identified	3—Departments Not specific as to high volume high risk areas (types of patients seen) Limited number of important aspect identified—does not cover scope
Indicators relating to the Q & A of the important aspects of care are identified	1—Department Documentation vs. clinically oriented indicators are monitored
Periodic assessment of the collected information is performed and measured against the pre-established criteria	3—Departments Data is collected just prior to QA Committee reporting date and does not cover entire quarter
Problems or opportunities to improve care are identified	1—Department Cases met criteria for each Indicator throughout the year
Action is taken as appropriate	1—Department Problems identified have not been resolved or not acted upon
The effectiveness of the action taken is evaluated	1—Department Indicators continue to be monitored with the same problems identified with no action taken
Reported through the channels established by the Hospital	1—Department Not consistent in reporting to QA Committee within designated time frame
There is evidence of the director's responsibility for and involvement in QA activities	1—Department The appraisal form or other QA reports do not reflect the Director's review of the info
The results of QA are used in continuing education of department members	2—Departments Topics for continuing education are not linked to QA results— Education is one action used to resolved problems
QA results are used to appraise the competence of those individuals within the department	5—Departments QA results are not being taken into consideration at the time of the employee's evaluation
New Indicators have been developed for 1988 if few problems were identified in 1987	2—Departments When problems are not identified through the monitoring process, this is a good indication that either criteria need to be revised or new areas can be monitored. *(continued)*

1987 Appraisal Evaluation Scoring Sheet (continued)

Quality Assurance Program Evaluation
Follow-Up

Department	April, 1991 Evaluation Results	May, 1991 Previous Action	Action Needed and Action to Date
Social Services	Evaluation of the quality assurance data that is collected is not done often enough.	QA committee approved that Social Services report three times a year instead of twice a year. The time frames for monitoring were revised.	Has not reported the results of monitoring activities as yet—Report due in August.
Dietary	Monitoring is not comprehensive. More indicators need to be developed and reported on a consistent basis—Lacks a planned and systematic process.	Along with the Director of Anesthesia, new indicators were developed to encompass the important aspects of care. Time frames were developed for monitoring.	Reported in May to QA committee on some of the indicators that were developed. Met with director in May to discuss how the data could be collected for all indicators developed.
Surgery	Consistent reporting of all indicators that are monitored is not performed or reported to the QA committee.	The Outpatient Head Nurse is collecting quality assurance data. QAP Committee approved that she be present at the QAP meetings to report Outpatient Surgery Quality Assurance.	Head Nurse is attending QA Committee and consistently reporting on the results of QA activities.
Laboratory	The same Indicators have been monitored for over a one year period with very few problems identified.	Examples of indicators were sent to the chief technician. She is in the process of developing some new indicators.	One new clinical indicator has been developed. Patient survey has been developed. Still need to replace indicators that are consistent achieving 100%.
Critical Care	Not all sections within the Department are reporting quality assurance in the proper format. Comprehensive reports are not being presented to the QA Committee per the reporting agenda.	Developed a reporting format for each section with separate indicators for each section.	Now reporting in the proper format. Presently developing clinically related indicators.

FIGURE A.2. *Form distributed among staff members responsible for departmental QA as a tool used to evaluate departmental quality assurance activities. The "1 2 3 4 5" rating system resembles that of the Joint Commission's accreditation survey. The second page is a tabulation of the rating scores of 13 departmental directors who completed the survey. The third page is the explanation of all low scores (scores of 3, 4, or 5). The fourth and final page contains documentation of the improvement of monitoring and evaluation in individual hospital departments.*
SOURCE: *Gail Bronswick, manager, professional services, Quality Healthcare Resources, Inc, a not-for-profit subsidiary of the Joint Commission, Oakbrook Terrace, IL.*

QA Program Evaluation 87/88 Consensus Rating Instrument

Rating—Definition of Compliance Score

1. *Substantial*—Full intent of standard met, with very minor exceptions
2. *Significant*—All major requirements met
3. *Partial*—Marginally meets all major requirements
4. *Minimal*—Minor expectations met, but doesn't address basic intent
5. *Non-compliance*—Not present at all; OR completely unresponsive to intent of standard

I. EVALUATION COMPONENT—STRUCTURE
   1. A current plan exists that delineates the QA program's objectives, organizational scope, review processes and the mechanicas for overseeing the effectiveness of QA activities.
      Comments: _____ 1 2 3 4 5
   2. Lines of authority and responsibility for carrying out QA activities are well delineated.
      Comments: _____ 1 2 3 4 5
   3. The existing committee structure facilitates efficient accomplishment of QA objectives.
      Comments: _____ 1 2 3 4 5
   4. The QA organizational structure promotes horizontal integration and communications concerning QA activities.
      Comments: _____ 1 2 3 4 5

II. EVALUATION COMPONENT—RESOURCE ALLOCATION AND SUPPORT
   1. The number and type of support staff devoted to quality assurance, utilization management, and risk management are adequate to insure maintenance of an ongoing monitoring and evaluation process.
      Comments: _____ 1 2 3 4 5
   2. QA program nonpersonnel resources (ie, materials, and equipment, including data systems) are sufficient to meet program objectives.
      Comments: _____ 1 2 3 4 5
   3. QA staff consistently provide needed advice and assistance to medical staff and hospital departments concerning QA reference materials.
      Comments: _____ 1 2 3 4 5

III. EVALUATION COMPONENT-PROCESS
   1. The QA program is comprehensive, including all clinical departments and all required medical staff QA functions.
      Comments: _____ 1 2 3 4 5
   2. The QA program is effective in generating, evaluating and reporting QA data in a easy to understand format.
      Comments: _____ 1 2 3 4 5
   3. QA indicators are objective, clinically valid and address significant aspects of care.
      Comments: _____ 1 2 3 4 5
   4. Routine and adequate documentation of QA activities is accomplished.
      Comments: _____ 1 2 3 4 5
   5. There is appropriate follow-up on identified problems/issues by involved departments and committees.
      Comments: _____ 1 2 3 4 5
   6. Medical staff, hospital department personnel and committees regularly report the results of activities to the Quality Assurance Committee as defined in the QA Plan.
      Comments: _____ 1 2 3 4 5

(continued)

QA Program Evaluation 87/88 Consensus Rating Instrument (continued)

7. Medical staff committees and hospital departmental personnel receive timely and useful feedback concerning reported QA activities.
   Comments: _____   1 2 3 4 5
8. The Board of Directors, through the Quality of Care Committee, receives regular reports of QA activities and mechanisms for identifying and resolving quality problems.
   Comments: _____   1 2 3 4 5
9. JCAHO standards have been identified and substantial compliance is evident as related to previous survey recommendations.
   Comments: _____   1 2 3 4 5

IV. EVALUATION COMPONENT—IMPACT
   1. QA monitoring activities have resulted in the identification and resolution of problems.
      Comments: _____   1 2 3 4 5
   2. The results of QA monitoring activities include improved patient outcomes.
      Comments: _____   1 2 3 4 5
   3. QA monitoring activities have led to improved clinical performance.
      Comments: _____   1 2 3 4 5
   4. QA information is used in medical staff credentialing and delineation of clinical privileges.
      Comments: _____   1 2 3 4 5
   5. The effectiveness of QA activities is evaluation at least annually at the department/committee level.
      Comments: _____   1 2 3 4 5
   6. Departments/committees implement appropriate QA program improvements based on the results of annual review.
      Comments: _____   1 2 3 4 5
   7. The overall effectiveness of the QA programs of the medical staff and hospital is evaluated annually.
      Comments: _____   1 2 3 4 5
   8. General medical staff/hospital improvements are implemented as appropriate based on the results of annual review.
      Comments: _____   1 2 3 4 5

Program Strengths: _____
Areas for Improvement: _____
Recommendations: _____

FIGURE A.3. *Consensus evaluation instrument with which key staff members can rate the effectiveness of the organization's QA program.*
SOURCE: *Wickemeier KM and Hamm M: The QA program evaluation: A powerful punch.* Journal of Quality Assurance *12(2):29, April/May/June 1990.*

Monitoring & Evaluation (M&E) Review System Program Evaluation Annual Report

Date: _____ Department/Service/Unit: _____

Person Responsible for M&E System: _____

Please evaluate your M&E System based on the following outline of the ten (10) key elements of an effective M&E Review System.

Elements of Monitoring & Evaluation System	Yes	No	N/A
I. Assignment of Responsibility			
A. The appropriate policy/procedure clearly assigns the responsibility for monitoring and evaluation to the unit/discipline chief?			
B. Department head's participation and responsibility is documented through: job description, performance evaluation, staff minutes, etc.			
C. Department head defines the responsibilities of others in the department and ensures that these responsibilities are fulfilled.			
D. Comments:			
II. Delineation of Scope of Care/Service			
A. Unit/discipline staff have clearly delineated the scope of care/services given by the department/unit?			
B. This delineation describes:			
1) Services/procedures provided			
2) Types of patients served			
3) Diagnosis/conditions treated			
4) Types of practitioners providing care			
5) Other:			
C. This delineation of scope of services is clearly documented in appropriate unit/department manual?			
D. Comments:			

(continued)

Monitoring & Evaluation (M&E) Review System Program Evaluation Annual Report (continued)

ELEMENTS OF MONITORING & EVALUATION SYSTEM	YES	NO	N/A
III. Identification of Important Aspects of Care A. Important aspects of care have been identified			
B. The monitoring & evaluation system is focused on the identified important aspects of care.			
C. The monitoring & evaluation system focuses on important aspects of care which:			
1) Occur frequently (high volume)			
2) Are of high risk (high risk)			
3) Historically have been problematic (problem prone)			
D. There is a link between the aspects of care included in the monitoring & evaluation system and the privileges granted by the department, as well as the duties delineated in performance evaluation programs.			
E. Comments:			
IV. Identification of Indicators A. For each important aspect of patient care, measurable indicators have been identified.			
B. The indicators developed include			
1) Process Indicators			
2) Outcome Indicators			
C. Indicators relevant to staff privileges or performance tasks are included in the monitoring & evaluation system.			
D. Data has been used for privileging or performance evaluations during the last year.			
E. For each indicator the following have been identified:			
1) Data sources			
2) Data collection method			
3) Frequency of data collection*			
F. Comments:			
V. Establish Criteria or Thresholds of Performance A. For each indicator, an evaluation threshold has been established (ie, a dividing line between performance that need not be reviewed further and performance that requires further evaluation).			
B. Comments:			

*Ideally, concurrent data collection takes place.

(continued)

Monitoring & Evaluation (M&E) Review System Program Evaluation Annual Report (continued)

Elements of Monitoring & Evaluation System	Yes	No	N/A
VI. Collection of Data			
A. Indicator data is regularly collected.			
B. Comparisons to the thresholds for evaluation are periodically or continuously made.			
C. Data collected outside the department is evaluated by your department.			
D. Comments:			
VII. Evaluation			
A. Evaluation of cumulative data is accomplished by qualified staff.			
B. During the past year cumulative data have indicated opportunities for improvement present.			
C. When data comparison shows the thresholds for evaluation have not been triggered, more detailed evaluation of each case takes place.			
D. Comments:			
VIII. Actions Taken to Improve Care/ IX. Assessment of Effectiveness of Actions/Documentation of Improvement			
A. During the last year, evaluations have concluded that care is acceptable and no further action was required:			

If YES, please list indicators: _____
_____
_____

B. During the last year, the following indicators have identified opportunities for improvement.

1)	Indicator:		
	Brief Description (who or what is expected to change):		
	Corrective Action Taken:		
	Continued Monitoring Indicates Problem Resolution? (circle one)	YES	NO
	Follow-up: When and how effectiveness of corrective action will be evaluated:		

(continued)

Monitoring & Evaluation (M&E) Review System Program Evaluation Annual Report (continued)

ELEMENTS OF MONITORING & EVALUATION SYSTEM

2) Indicator:

Brief Description (who or what is expected to change):

Corrective Action Taken:

Continued Monitoring Indicates Problem Resolution? (circle one)   YES   NO

Follow-up: When and how effectiveness of corrective action will be evaluated:

3) Indicator:

Brief Description (who or what is expected to change):

Corrective Action Taken:

Continued Monitoring Indicates Problem Resolution? (circle one)   YES   NO

Follow-up: When and how effectiveness of corrective action will be evaluated:

4) Indicator:

Brief Description (who or what is expected to change):

Corrective Action Taken:

Continued Monitoring Indicates Problem Resolution? (circle one)   YES   NO

Follow-up: When and how effectiveness of corrective action will be evaluated:

5) Indicator:

Brief Description (who or what is expected to change):

Corrective Action Taken:

Continued Monitoring Indicates Problem Resolution? (circle one)   YES   NO

Follow-up: When and how effectiveness of corrective action will be evaluated:

(continued)

Monitoring & Evaluation (M&E) Review System Program Evaluation Annual Report (continued)

Elements of Monitoring & Evaluation System	Yes	No	N/A
X. Communication of Monitoring & Evaluation (M&E) Information A. The results of M&E are reported, discussed, and documented in staff meeting minutes.			
B. M&E reports are submitted to the Quality Assurance Department.			
C. M&E reports are also submitted to (please list):			
D. Results of M&E are communicated for use in the periodic reappraisal of those who are granted clinical privileges and in the performance evaluation programs of other health care providers.			
E. Comments:			

Annual Revision	Yes	No	N/A
A. The present monitoring and evaluation system needs to be updated/ revised in the following areas: 1) Assignment of responsibility			
2) Delineation of scope of care			
3) Identification of important aspects of care			
4) Indicators			
5) Thresholds for evaluation			
6) Data collection/organization			
7) Evaluation of care			
8) Actions Taken			
9) Assessment of effectiveness of actions			
10) Communication of information			
B. Please indicate revisions to be made and target date for each:			
C. In determining need for revisions did you take into account: 1) Facility Evaluations/Studies			
2) Utilization Review Findings			
3) Committee Findings			
4) External Review Findings			
5) Previous QA Findings			
D. What is the most positive impact on patient care your monitoring & evaluation system has had during the last year?			

Figure A.4. Form to help evaluate a health care organization's monitoring and evaluation activities. Appropriate for use by governing boards, this form employs a simple yes/no format.
Source: Gary Pomeroy, surveyor, Hospital Accreditation Program, Joint Commission, Oakbrook Terrace, IL.

Completed Assessment Matrix for State Psychiatric Hospital

Assessment Questions	Credentialing/ licensure, certification/ registration[1]	Privileging (appraisal/ reappraisal)	Performance appraisal	Patient care monitoring (individual case review)	Treatment plan review	Special treatment procedures monitoring[2]	Dietary (food acceptance studies)	Safety	Infection control	Medical support services[3]
1. Is the function performed by an individual or committee?	Comm.	Comm.	Ind.	Ind.	Team	Ind.	Ind.	Comm.	Comm.	Comm.
2. Who is routinely responsible for the function?	Chair of priv. com. med. staff	Chair of priv. com. med. staff	Unit chief	Disc. chief	Team leader	DDC	Dietitian	DDA	Nurse	DDC
3. Is there a written description or procedure for the function?	Yes	Yes	Yes	Yes	No*	Yes	Yes	No*	Yes	Yes
4. What data sources are used to perform this function?	Transcripts, licenses, diplomas, application form	Work sample, QA findings, supervisory report	Intuition	Case record, oral presentation	Case record, oral presentation	Daily reports	Patient interview, waste review	Observation	Bacterial sampling	Record inspection
5. Are preestablished clinically valid criteria used?	Yes	Yes	No*	No*	No*	No*	No*	Yes	Yes	Yes
6. If a purpose of the function is to identify problems, are important problems identified?	N/A	Yes / Yes	No* / No*	Yes / No*	Yes / No*	Yes / No*	Yes / Yes	Yes / Yes	Yes / Yes	Yes / Yes
7. Have actions been taken to resolve identified problems or to improve care?	Yes	No	No	Yes	Yes	Yes	No	No		
8. Does the responsible individual or committee recommend or implement action?	Rec.	Rec.	Rec.	Rec.	Impl.	Impl.	Impl.	Both	Rec.	Impl.
9. Is there monitoring to determine effectiveness of action?	No*	No*	No*	Yes	Yes	Yes	No*	Yes	Yes	Yes
10. To whom are the results of the function reported? With whom are they shared?	Dir. / DQA, DDC, disc. chief	Dir. / DQA disc. chief	Not* shared / Payroll	DQA / DDC, disc. chief	Not* shared / Not* shared	Not* shared / DQA	DQA / DQA	DDA / DQA, gov. body	Infec. control comm. / DQA, DDC	Pharm comm. / DQA, DDC
11. Is the function evaluated routinely?	No*	No*	No*	No*	No*	No*	No*	No*	No*	No*

DDA = Deputy director administration
DDC = Deputy director clinical
DQA = Director of quality assurance
OCC = Quality control committee
*This component should be conducted, but is not.

(continued)

Completed Assessment Matrix for State Psychiatric Hospital (continued)

Rehabilitation support services[4]	Utilization review	Referral monitoring	Program evaluation	Optional support services[5]	Professional growth and development	Employee orientation	Research	Incident report	Support services	Mortality	Patient records
Comm.		★	Ind.	★	Dept.	Dept.		Comm.	★	Comm.	Comm.
Unit chiefs	DDC	★	Dir. prog. eval.	★	Dir. ed. & trng.	Dir. ed. & trng.	Research review board	DDC	★	DDC	Dir. med. rec.
Yes	Yes	★	Yes	★	Yes	Yes	Yes	Yes	★	No*	No*
Record super. report, work sample	Medical record	★	Plan goals & obj. log MIS	★	Satisfactory process logs, audit	Logs, attend-ance sheet	Proposal protocol monitoring forms	Incident report, patient record	★	Autopsy, patient record	Patient record
Yes	Yes	★	Yes	★	No*	Yes	Yes	No*	★	No*	No*
Yes	Yes	★	No*	★	No*	No*	No*	Yes	★	Yes	Yes
Yes	No*		No*		No*	No*	No*	Yes		No*	Yes
Impl.	Rec.	★	Rec.	★	Impl.	Impl.	Rec.	Rec.	★	Rec.	Impl.
No*	Yes	★	No*	★	Yes	No*	Yes	No*	★	No*	No*
DQA	Comm.	★	Plan comm.	★	DDA	Not* shared	Dir. of research	QCC, gov. body	★	QCC, DDC	DQA, DDC
Not* shared	DQA, DDC	★	DQA, unit chiefs	★	DQA			DQA, board of visitors	★	DQA	Dir. med. rec.
No*	No*	★	Yes	★	Yes	No*	No*	No*	★	No*	No*

[1]Indicate appropriate process for each discipline.
[2]Monitoring of restraints, seclusion, ECT, psychosurgery, behavior modification, research, drugs (schedule 11), aversive therapy.
[3]Monitoring of anesthesia, radiology, pharmacy.
[4]Monitoring of speech, hearing, occupational therapy, educational services, vocational rehabilitation, activity therapy.
[5]Monitoring of volunteers, community education, outreach, pastoral counseling.

FIGURE A.5. Matrix (in this case, already completed) to help evaluate the hospital's QA program.

QA Status Report to QA Committee

*Exception Report
(Only those departments
with QA problems are listed)*

Date: _____

Department	Delinquent (# of Months)	Minutes Do Not Meet Standards	QA Plan and/or Systems Inadequate

Problems/Action/Follow-up Do Not Exist	Significant Quality of Care Problems and Actions	QA Coordinator/Chairperson/Admin. Action to Correct Deficiencies

FIGURE A.6. *Organizationwide form to record deficiencies in departmental QA activities or plans.* SOURCE: *Dunn C: Communicating quality to the board.* Journal of Quality Assurance 10(5):24, Dec/Jan 1989.

Summary Information on Monitoring & Evaluation of Quality & Appropriateness of Patient Care and Clinical Performance

HOSPITAL _____DATE _____

PATIENT PROFILE DATA

Please list the following, as applicable, for the most recent 12 months:

The five most common
    principal diagnoses for adult medical (nonsurgical, nonOB) inpatients and outpatients
    principal diagnoses for pediatric inpatients and outpatients
    principal nonOB, nonGYN surgical procedures for inpatients and outpatients
    principal gynecological surgical procedures for inpatients and outpatients
    nonsurgical invasive procedures for inpatients and outpatients

Number of obstetrical patients delivered:

Number spontaneous _____   Number C-sections: elective primary _____

Number induced   _____   elective repeat _____

Number forceps   _____   unplanned   _____

Number live births _____ Number premature/immature _____ Number fetal deaths _____

(continued)

Summary Information on Monitoring & Evaluation of Quality & Appropriateness of Patient Care and Clinical Performance (continued)

Please list for each of the following departments or services, as applicable to this hospital, the important aspects of patient care and clinical performance that were *monitored and evaluated for quality and appropriateness* within the past 12 months: Family Practice, Medicine, Obstetrics-Gynecology, Pediatrics, Psychiatry, Surgery, Anesthesia, Diagnostic Radiology, Emergency, Hospital Sponsored Ambulatory Care (including come-and-go surgery), Nuclear Medicine, Pathology and Medical Laboratory, Radiation Oncology, Rehabilitation, Respiratory Care, Special Care Units (MS.6.1.1 and corresponding standard in each support service).

SURGICAL CASE REVIEW (most recent 12 months)

Number of operations with tissue specimens _____
   Of these, the number not justified by the pathology report* _____
      Of these, the number subsequently justified by peer review _____
Number of operations without tissue specimens _____
   Of these, the number not justified by written screening criteria* _____
      Of these, the number subsequently justified by peer review _____
Number of non-surgical invasive procedures _____
   Of these, the number not meeting written screening criteria* _____
      Of these, the number subsequently justified by peer review _____
*Please attach copies of the pathology criteria for referring cases to peer review and of the screening criteria for the three most commonly performed non-tissue procedures and the three most common non-surgical invasive procedures.

Enter any explanatory comments relative to surgical case review information:

DRUG USAGE EVALUATION (most recent 12 months)

List the six most commonly prescribed classes of drugs in this hospital, exclusive of laxatives, decongestants, topical agents, IV solutions, nutrients:

_____   _____
_____   _____
_____   _____

Please list below the classes of drugs or specific drugs included in DUE in the past 12 months, indicating which uses were evaluated (Th = therapeutic, Pr = prophylactic, Em = empirical), the number of cases included and the departments and services:

Class of drug/specific drug	Th	Pr	Em	# Cases	Departments and Services
_____	__	__	__	_____	_____
_____	__	__	__	_____	_____
_____	__	__	__	_____	_____
_____	__	__	__	_____	_____
_____	__	__	__	_____	_____
_____	__	__	__	_____	_____
_____	__	__	__	_____	_____

Please attach copies of the criteria that were used in the two most recently concluded DUEs along with summary data on the findings.

(continued)

Summary Information on Monitoring & Evaluation of Quality & Appropriateness of Patient Care and Clinical Performance (continued)

BLOOD USAGE REVIEW (most recent 12 months)

Please complete the following table, excluding blood used in cardiac surgery cases:

	# cases transfused	# screened by written criteria*	# failing screen	# justified by peer review
Whole blood	_____	_____	_____	_____
Packed red cells	_____	_____	_____	_____
Fresh frozen plasma	_____	_____	_____	_____
Platelet concentrate	_____	_____	_____	_____
_____	_____	_____	_____	_____
_____	_____	_____	_____	_____
_____	_____	_____	_____	_____

*Please attach a copy of the criteria used to screen appropriateness of transfusion of whole blood and all listed components and derivatives.

What is the C/T ratio? _____
Number of verified transfusion reactions in past 12 months: _____
Briefly describe the most important improvement in transfusion therapy in the past 12 months:

PHARMACY AND THERAPEUTICS FUNCTION

Number of verified untoward drug reactions in the past 12 months: _____
Number of bleeding episodes from use of anticoagulants in past 12 months: _____
Please attach a copy of the guidelines for identifying untoward drug reactions and a copy of the medical staff's definition of significant untoward drug reaction.

Kindly provide the following information:

1. Briefly describe the mechanism in this hospital which assures the same level of quality of patient care by all individuals with clinical privileges, within medical staff departments, across departments/services, and between members and nonmembers of the medical staff who have delineated clinical privileges (MS.3.11, AMH 1988, p 119).

2. Briefly describe the mechanism in this hospital which assures that all individuals with clinical privileges provide services within the scope of privileges granted (MS.4.1.3, AMH 1988, p 119).

Please attach a copy of the most recent annual evaluation of the objectives, scope, organization, and effectiveness of the quality assurance program (QA.4.5, *AMH* 1988, p. 238).

FIGURE A.7. *Adjunct to an annual QA evaluation form. The first two pages help show whether monitored aspects of care address the most prevalent procedures performed and the most frequently prescribed potent drugs. The form may also indicate that monitored indicators are not meaningful (if few deviations were flagged by them) or that peer review is superficial (if almost all variations are justified). The question asking for a description of the most important improvement in the past 12 months highlights the expectation that monitoring and evaluation should lead to improvements. Most of the third page requests information on appointment, reappointment, and practitioner privileging.*

Quality Assurance Program Assessment

This assessment has been designed for you to evaluate our Quality Assurance Program. As you know, Quality Assurance is only as effective as we make it.

Please place a "✔" in the "Yes"/"No" columns with explanations, suggestions of who, what, where, and when in the "Comment" section.

A. Does the Quality Assurance Plan:

	Yes	No	Comments
1. Refer to the organization's philosophy?			
2. Refer to the organizations goals//objectives?			
3. Describe the purpose of the Quality Assurance program?			
4. Clearly define its goals/objectives?			
5. Define the program's scope including integration with hospital quality assurance and medical quality assurance programs?			
6. Address authority?			
7. Identify person(s) (position) responsible for coordinating the program?			
8. Describe the Quality Assurance committee: a. purpose/functions? b. membership? c. chairperson?			
9. Identify committees interfacing with Quality Assurance Committee?			
10. Describe a monitoring approach (i.e., problem-focused)?			
11. Delineate lines of communicating?			
12. Address confidentiality?			
13. Include a plan for periodic evaluation?			

B. As a result of Quality Assurance efforts, do you think:

	Yes	No	Comments
1. You appropriately utilize standard(s) established by: a. Nursing Division/Department(s)?			
b. ANA?			
c. JCAH?			
d. State/National Government?			
2. Your practice of nursing has improved?			
3. Your documentation has improved?			

(continued)

Quality Assurance Program Assessment (continued)

	Yes	No	Comments
4. Patient care has become more cost effective?			
5. Patient satisfaction has increased?			
6. Nurses' job satisfaction has increased?			
7. Staff performance appraisals are more accurate?			
8. Your time and involvement is worthwhile?			
9. Malpractice liability has decreased?			
10. Continuing education programs are more relevant?			

C. ADDITIONAL COMMENTS:

Nursing Unit _____

Name (optional) _____

FIGURE A.8. *Form designed to help evaluate the nursing QA program.*
SOURCE: *Meisenheimer CG:* Quality Assurance: A Complete Guide to Effective Programs. *Rockville, MD: Aspen Publishers, 1985, pp 76-77.*

Questionnaire: Evaluation of QA Activities

Use the questionnaire below to assess how well your nursing department makes effective use of QA activities. The questionnaire lists 21 department functions. Consider how each may be related to your QA program in terms of:

- *Topics. Which nursing department functions provide problems that need to be monitored via QA studies?*
- *Criteria. Which functions provide criteria for QA studies, or are themselves guided by QA criteria?*
- *Data. Which functions feed data into QA studies?*
- *Actions. Which functions are the vehicles for taking corrective action? And which might be significantly affected by QA study findings?*

Circle the dots in the columns at the right that apply. Any dots that remain uncircled represent areas of unexplored opportunity for interrelating nursing activities and QA.

Are You Interrelating Nursing Activities and QA?

Nursing Care Activities	QA Functions Topics	Criteria	Data	Actions
Infection control	•	•	•	•
Staff development	•	•	•	•
Nursing unit rounds	•	•	•	•
Nursing practice standards	•	•	•	•
Nursing service standards	•	•	•	•
Department policies/procedures	•	•	•	•
Incident reports	•	•	•	•
Safety/risk management	•	•	•	•
Liability claims	•	•	•	•
Performance appraisal	•	•	•	•
Care conferences	•	•	•	•
Committee meetings	•	•	•	•
Cost containment	•	•	•	•
Accreditation reports	•	•	•	•
Resources management	•	•	•	•
Nursing care plans	•	•	•	•
Discharge planning	•	•	•	•
Patient education	•	•	•	•
Suggestion boxes	•	•	•	•
Staff newsletter	•	•	•	•
Nursing research	•	•	•	•
Budget setting	•	•	•	•
Strategic planning	•	•	•	•

Now that you've completed the questionnaire, use a blank page to summarize your findings and to discover opportunities for interrelating nursing activities and quality assurance.

- *Look down the first column for uncircled dots. Which activities could provide study topics? List them in order of priority.*
- *Look down the second column for uncircled dots. Which activities could employ or provide QA study criteria? List them in order of priority.*
- *Look down the third column. Which activities could produce or could utilize study data?*
- *Look down the fourth column. Which activities could be better used for QA study actions?*

FIGURE A.9. *A creative format to evaluate the depth and breadth of a nursing QA program.*
SOURCE: *Adapted from Nursing Quality Assurance Management Learning System:* Workbook for Nursing Quality Assurance Committee Members: General Practice in Acute Care Hospitals. *American Nurses' Association and Sutherland Learning Associates, Inc, 1985.*

Quality Assurance Program Annual Evaluation

SUMMARY OF COMPLIANCE WITH HOSPITAL CRITERIA
1990–1991

List below the most important improvements in patient care that have resulted directly from the activities of the QA Program in the past 12 months.

	PERCENTAGE OF COMPLIANCE		
CRITERION	1982	1983	CHANGE (IN %)
Justified admissions	85	95	+ 10
Presence of indications for blood transfusion	75	85	+ 10
Absence of unjustified length of stay	60	75	+ 15
Absence of surgical wound infections	90	95	+ 5
Preadmission screening in elective surgery	55	75	+ 20
Third-party payer claims accepted as submitted	80	90	+ 10

FIGURE A.10. *Central to the annual evaluation of the QA program is evaluation of improvements brought by quality assurance.*
SOURCE: *Adapted from Carroll JG:* Restructuring Hospital Quality Assurance: The New Guide for Health Care Providers. *Homewood, IL: Dow Jones-Irwin, 1984, p 125.*

Nursing Quality Assessment Program Evaluation 1991–92

Unit Based Committees: Unit Trends in Departmentwide Indicators:

Indicator	Summarize Your Unit's Trends for 1988–89	What Unit Actions Were Taken	Effect of Action
Patient Falls			
Medication Errors			
Use of Med Inc Form			
Narcotic Sign-out			
Nursing Process			
Code 99			
Nursing Documentation			
Transfer Summary			
Nosocomial Infection			
IV Phlebitis			
Pressure Sores			
Other			

Figure A.11. *Form to stimulate evaluation of the QA program through documenting QA actions taken to improve care and effects of those actions.*
Source: *Day G: Evaluating a nursing QA program.* Journal of Quality Assurance 12(3):24, Jul/ Aug 1990.

Hospital Staff Satisfaction with Department of Quality Assurance Consultation

Date: _____

Department/Person Consulted: _____

MONITOR TITLE:
Review of Appropriateness of Consultation from QA Department QA Consultant: _____

1. Was the consultation initiated by you and/or QA staff:
   ☐ a) QA staff
   ☐ b) myself
   ☐ c) others: _____
   If you made the initial contact, was response from personnel in the QA Department timely, courteous, and appropriate?
   ☐ Yes   ☐ No

2. Was there a preestablished reason or agenda for the consultation?
   ☐ Yes   ☐ No
   Comments: _____

3. Did the QA person help you with your identified issue or problem in the following ways?
   ☐ a) Develop quality assurance plan
   ☐ b) Develop quality assurance monitor
   ☐ c) Trend quality assurance monitor
   ☐ d) Analyze data and make recommendations
   ☐ e) Identify systems problems or interdepartmental monitor topics
   ☐ f) Other: _____
   ☐ g) Present a QA educational program
   ☐ h) Summarize a monitor report/annual QA report

4. Did you receive clear, concise minutes of each of your consultations?
   ☐ Yes   ☐ No

5. Were the minutes helpful in clarifying what should be done or who was supposed to do it?
   ☐ Yes   ☐ No

6. How would you rate the overall assistance you received from the QA person you worked with?
   ☐ a) Extremely helpful and thorough
   ☐ b) Helpful but confusing
   ☐ c) Not that helpful to me
   ☐ d) I need help but the QA consultant does not meet my needs

7. I would like to have the QA consultant improve in the following ways: (Please be open about your comments.) _____

8. Did you think the QA consultation helped you to identify QA monitors that helped you evaluate the following: (check all that apply)
   ☐ a) Effectiveness   ☐ Yes   ☐ No
   ☐ b) Efficiency   ☐ Yes   ☐ No
   ☐ c) Accessibility   ☐ Yes   ☐ No
   ☐ d) Acceptability   ☐ Yes   ☐ No
   ☐ e) Competency   ☐ Yes   ☐ No

9. Did the QA consultant help you review the following: (check all that apply)
   ☐ a) Clinical or service outcomes of QA   ☐ Yes   ☐ No
   ☐ b) Management outcomes of QA   ☐ Yes   ☐ No

FIGURE A.12. *Questionnaire used to survey the satisfaction of clinical staff members with the services and consultations they receive from the organization's QA department.*
SOURCE: *Martin NS: A QA monitor for the QA department.* Journal of Quality Assurance 9(4):25, *Fall 1987.*

Quality Assurance Program Evaluation Questionnaire

Please answer each question using rating scale noted below, and please explain any *ratings of Disagree or Strongly Disagree in Comments below.*

Person completing questionnaire: _____

From whom do you receive regular reports/data regarding Quality Assurance: _____

	Strongly Agree	Agree	Disagree	Strongly Disagree	No Opinion	Not Applicable
1. I regularly use QA data in decision-making. Comment: _____						
2. QA data is generally: · Reliable · Received in a timely manner · In an acceptable format · Of an acceptable amount such that it can be used for my purposes. Comment: _____						
3. My department has adequate resources to accomplish quality assurance functions. List the estimated work hours devoted to QA activities per month: _____						
4. I feel I am able to receive helpful technical assistance as needed for designing/revising my QA program. Comment: _____						
5. I feel that my current clinical indicators adequately reflect significant dimensions of care provided in my area. Comment: _____						
6. In the past year we have documented that patient care has improved as a direct result of QA activities. List how many such instance are documented: _____						
7. Recommendations from QA activities in my area are consistently acted upon or implemented. Comment: _____						
8. I would be less informed from an objective perspective regarding the quality of services in my area if QA monitoring were eliminated. Comment: _____						

Thank you for your time in completing this questionnaire.
Please return completed form to: _____

by: _____
Date

FIGURE A.13. A survey instrument asking department leaders for their opinions on the effectiveness of their own department's QA. "Even the best QA programs require periodic review to refocus and correct ailing subsystems . . . and to direct optimal QA resource allocation," according to administrators at the hospital that created this form.
SOURCE: Wickemeier KM, Hamm M: The QA program evaluation: A powerful punch. Journal of Quality Assurance *12(2): 30, April/May/June 1990.*

Nursing Quality Assurance Program Evaluation 1988–89
Staff Nurse Questionnaire

INITIAL DATA:

Shift: ☐ 7–3   ☐ Part time   Length of time at BSH: Degree obtained:
      ☐ 3–11   ☐ Full time   ☐ Less than 1 year   ☐ 2 – 5 years   ☐ RN   ☐ BSN
      ☐ 11–7   ☐ Pool   ☐ 1 – 2 years   ☐ Over 5 years ☐ ADN   ☐ MS

I FEEL NURSING QUALITY ASSURANCE ACTIVITIES:	TRUE	FALSE
• Are something I know nothing about.	☐	☐
• Are for a Quality Assurance Coordinator only.	☐	☐
• Should be handled by a unit-level coordinator.	☐	☐
• Are for the supervisory level of nursing.	☐	☐
• Do not involve me at all.	☐	☐
• Are a waste of time.	☐	☐
• Are primarily used to meet accreditation requirements.	☐	☐
• Are part of my daily nursing activities.	☐	☐
• Are well communicated to the staff on the unit I work.	☐	☐
• Provide an opportunity for me to have a say in changing my nursing practice.	☐	☐
• Have made some changes that have improved patient care.	☐	☐
• Are something I would like to know more about.	☐	☐
• Look at the important things that I do as a nurse.	☐	☐
• Are well understood by the staff nurses.	☐	☐

IN THE LAST YEAR I HAVE BEEN INVOLVED IN THE FOLLOWING ACTIVITIES:	(Check all that pertain)
• Reviewing the nursing care given by other registered nurses.	☐
• Developing standards of nursing care.	☐
• Serving on a unit-based QA committee.	☐
• Assisting in data collection for a nursing QA activity.	☐
• Using the results of quality assurance improvements in the delivery of my nursing care.	☐

Please answer yes or no and rank these eight activities as to their importance in the role of the registered nurse by numbering them from one to eight by importance (one being the most important). Put the number on the space prior to the activity.

IF I COULD, I WOULD . . .	YES	NO
___ • Spend more time teaching patient and/or families.	☐	☐
___ • Involve patient in planning their care.	☐	☐
___ • Improve skills in performing nursing care procedures.	☐	☐
___ • Spend more time planning patient's care.	☐	☐
___ • Write nursing care standards for my specialty area.	☐	☐
___ • Participate in reviewing the nursing care given by other nurses.	☐	☐
___ • Spend more time doing discharge planning for my patient.	☐	☐
___ • Be an active member on a quality assurance unit committee.	☐	☐

Please write any additional comments or suggestions on the back. Thank you for your assistance in this evaluation process. We hope to make Nursing Quality Assurance an even more meaningful part of your activities as we structure our program for 1989-90!

FIGURE A.14. *Questionnaire for gathering information on nurses' perceptions of and involvement with quality assurance activities.*
SOURCE: *Day G: Evaluating a nursing QA program.* Journal of Quality Assurance 12(3):25, Jul/ Aug 1990.

**Staff Perception Questionnaire
RE: Quality Assurance**

1. What does quality assurance mean to you? _____

    _____

    _____

    _____

2. Does quality assurance apply to your job? How is it used in your department/service? _____

    _____

    _____

    _____

3. Have quality assurance activities improved patient care or services in the past year? Please explain your answer. _____

    _____

    _____

    _____

4. Do you feel quality assurance committees and staff members have supported your efforts to enhance quality care and services? Have you received helpful suggestions for resolving identified problems from the quality assurance committees and staff members? Give examples of support or lack of support. _____

    _____

    _____

    _____

5. What do you think would improve the quality of patient care (eg, new activities or programs)?

    _____

    _____

    _____

    _____

6. In your opinion, in what areas do quality assurance groups and leaders need to improve? What changes should they make? _____

    _____

    _____

    _____

7. What aspects of quality assurance related to patient care do you feel are the strongest? _____

    _____

    _____

    _____

FIGURE A.15. Questionnaire for staff to record their perceptions about quality assurance.

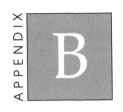

APPENDIX

B

Using Practitioner-Specific QA Results in Renewal/Revision of Clinical Privileges and Reappointment to the Medical Staff

QA activities may provide objective data (including findings of monitoring and evaluation, utilization review, infection control, and risk management) that are relevant to determinations about the renewal/revision of clinical privileges and individual practitioners' reappointment to the medical staff. In so doing, the organization can look at such things as the physician's complication rates, performance related to key indicators, drug prescribing practices, and number of complex procedures performed (to help assess whether the number was sufficient to maintain clinical competence). If these data are gathered and maintained for each practitioner in the QA process, they should be available for use in the clearly defined mechanisms used to authorize a practitioner's scope of clinical practice.

Joint Commission standards require that relevant findings from quality assurance activities be considered as part of the reappraisal process for reappointment to the medical staff and for the renewal/revision of clinical privileges, and in the process used to appraise the competence of all those individuals not permitted by the hospital to practice independently.

The focus of using QA results in clinical privileging and reappointment to the medical staff is to provide objective data on all practitioners, the vast majority of whom are meeting, if not exceeding, standards. Practitioner-specific data lend confidence and objectivity to reappointment decisions; they are not gathered in order to punish practitioners. In those few instances where quality data identify physicians in need of assistance, this information should be used in directing efforts to improve physician practice through educational efforts and/or improvement in clinical support systems. Only as a last resort should a facility consider curtailing or removing privileges.

Any practitioner-specific QA data should, of course, be treated as highly confidential and be kept in credentials files (designated as necessary to ensure protection under applicable state law).

Well-designed forms such as physician QA profiles provide a structure for including objective, physician-specific QA data in performance-based reappointment. Figure B.1. is an open-ended form for listing various types of indicator rates for a practitioner. Figures B.2. through B.4. are examples of physician QA profiles that are consulted during reappraisal.

Some of the forms in this appendix give only numerators (eg, "number of deficiencies") without denominators (eg, total number of the physician's patients for whom the event of interest could have occurred by reason of their having the condition or procedure the indicator is monitoring). Denominator data are often overlooked, but may be important in assessing the significance of the data during the reappraisal.

In general, any form that includes physician-specific monitoring and evaluation results can be looked at during reappraisal. Thus, forms in the evaluation chapter are especially good for this purpose (eg, see Figures 7.N. through 7.T.). Figures B.5. and B.6. are physician-specific summaries of indicator data. Figure B.5. displays a particular physician's level of activity at the hospital and how the physician compares to the hospital mean for performance indicators.

Figures B.7. and B.8. are recommendation forms (on which the decision is written whether to grant reappointment).

Individual Reappointment Profile

NAME: DEPARTMENT: SECTION: ID #:

TOPICS/INSTRUCTIONS	RESULTS	PATTERNS
Transfers to psychiatric and rehab units *Instruction:* Give total number, rate	9 cases; 4%	Physician's rate is same as in previous year and is below the 5.5% rate for dept.
Admission denials *Instruction:* Give total number, rate	18 cases; 8.3%	Physician's rate (8.3%) is second highest in dept.
CONTINUED STAYS Total inpatient days	1140 days	Physician's inpatient days decreased by 5% from previous year
Average LOS	7.1 days	Physician's LOS is above dept average of 6.4 days but has decreased from 8.4 days in previous year.
Stays in excess of outlier threshold *Instruction:* Give number of cases, total days	17 cases 64 days	No comparative data from previous year; physician ranks 4th in dept in number of outlier cases.
Stays denied reimbursement *Instruction:* Give number of cases denied reimbursement, total days	2 cases 13 days	Physician had no denials during previous year.

(continued)

Individual Reappointment Profile (continued)

NAME:	DEPARTMENT:	SECTION:	ID #:

TOPICS/INSTRUCTIONS	RESULTS	PATTERNS
Stays in special care unit *Instruction:* Give number of cases, average LOS, number of cases exceeding 8 days	*Total:* 10 cases *Avg LOS:* 4 days *Excessive stays:* 1 case	Physician's LOS (4 days) is above dept average of 3.2 days.
Short stays (1,2,3 days) *Instruction:* Give number of cases, number of cases readmitted within 30 days	17 cases 2 readmitted	No current comparative data available.

SURGICAL INVASIVE PROCEDURES
Procedures performed
Instruction: Give breakdown by type of procedure
	Total: 10 procedures
	Procedure
	  Gastroscopy: 4
	  Colonoscopy: 2
	  Biopsy: 4
		Physician's procedures increased from a total of 4 during previous year.

DRUG ORDERS All drug orders *Instruction:* Give total number of services ordered, total costs, average cost/case	*Total services ordered:* 6440 *Total costs:* $42,175 *Average cost/case:* $238	Total costs for physician increased from $22,140 in previous year. Physician's average cost/case exceeds dept avg of $188.

Orders for specific meds
Instruction: Give total number of orders, costs for:
  -antihypertensives
  -anticoagulants
  -aminoglycosides
  -psychotropics
  -cephalosporins
	Antihypertensives: 19 cases, $12,040;
	Anticoagulants: 0 cases, $0;
	Aminoglycosides: 14 cases, $2,450;
	Psychotropics: 4 cases, $780
	Cephalosporins: 12 cases, $6,780
		No previous data available; physician's current average costs for antihypertensives, cephalosporins exceeds dept average of $4,215 per case.

Orders for nonformulatory drugs *Instruction:* Give breakdown by type of drug	0	N/A
Orders for IV solutions *Instruction:* Give total number of services, total costs	*Services:* 915 *Cost:* $8,510	Physician's orders for services, costs decreased from a total of 1214 services, $11,510 in previous year.
BLOOD USE Total units ordered/transfused	*Ordered:* 24 *Transfused:* 18	No trend data available
BLOOD USE Total orders for emergency crossmatches	0	N/A
THERAPEUTIC PROCEDURES Orders for Dx imaging *Instruction:* Give total number of services ordered, total costs, average cost/case	*Total services:* 1040 *Total costs:* $29,114 *Average cost/case:* $152	Physician's costs decreased from a total of $36,450 in previous year. Physician's current average cost/case is below dept avg of $210. *(continued)*

Individual Reappointment Profile (continued)

NAME: DEPARTMENT: SECTION: ID #:

TOPICS/INSTRUCTIONS	RESULTS	PATTERNS

Orders for specific types of imaging studies
Instruction: Give total number services, % of admissions receiving service for following:
    chest x-rays
    portables
    special invasive studies
    CT
	Chests: 595 services
	    98% of admits
	Portables: 140 services
	    7% of admits
	Invasives: 36 services
	    12% of admits
	CTs: 0 services
	    0% of admits
		Physician's orders for chests increased from previous year (380, 9.9% of admits); order for portables decreased (220, 34% of admits); orders for invasives increased (20, 8% of admits); orders for CT were the same.

Orders for clinical laboratory services *Instruction:* Give total number of services, costs, average services per stay	*Total services:* 3613 *Total costs:* $86,750 *Avg. services per stay:* 13.5	Physician's total lab costs are highest in dept; his average number of services per stay exceeds dept avg of 8.5.

Orders for specific types of clinical lab studies
Instruction: Give total number of services, average services per stay for: -ESR
        -cardiac/enzymes
        -protimes
	ESR: 380 services
	    4.3/stay
	Cardiac/enzymes: 1125 services
	        5.7/stay
	Protimes: 915 services
	        8.0/stay
		No comparative data available.

STAT chem orders *Instruction:* Give total number of services ordered, % of all chem services ordered STAT	689 services 19% of all chem services	No previous data available; physician's percentage of chem services ordered STAT exceeds dept avg of 17.7%.
Orders for aerosol therapy *Instruction:* Give total number of services, costs	*Services:* 512 *Costs:* $5,815	No comparative data currently available.
DOCUMENTATION Delinquent records *Instruction:* Give total number of records delinquent, % of discharges	39 records 10% of discharges	Physician's percentage of delinquent records exceeds hospital average of 12%.

FIGURE B.1. An open-ended form to list a practitioner's rate of compliance with indicators as well as related patterns of care (ie, comparisons to his or her historical performance and to other staff physicians).
SOURCE: *Joseph ED, Devet C, Dehn TG:* The Monitoring Sourcebook, Volume 3: Physician Practice Monitors. *Chicago: Care Communications, 1986, pp 268-271.*

QRM Summary for Reappointment

Physician Code #: _____ Service Dept: _____

Staff Status: _____ Reappointment due (date): _____

Performance Profile (Time Period _____)

QUALITY AND APPROPRIATENESS MONITORING

# discharges screened	_____
# cases referred for peer review	___/___%
service average	___/___%
# patients with APOs	___/___%
service average	___/___%
# of patients with APOs severity $\geq$ 3	___/___%
service average	___/___%
# of APOs with (+) SOC (Code 1,2)	___/___%
service average	___/___%
# of APOs with ($\pm$) SOC (Code 3)	___/___%
service average	___/___%
# of APOs with (−) SOC (Code 4)	___/___%
service average	___/___%

INVASIVE PROCEDURE/SURGICAL CASE REVIEW

Procedures performed (total)	_____
service average/physician	_____

#	Procedure	#	Procedure
	_____		_____
	_____		_____
	_____		_____
	_____		_____
	_____		_____

# tissue reviews	_____
# questionable	_____
# inappropriate	_____
# nondiagnostic/normal tissue reviews	_____
# questionable	_____
# inappropriate	_____
# non-tissue reviews	_____
# questionable	_____
# inappropriate	_____

TRANSFUSION REVIEW

# units T&C	_____
service average	_____
# units T&S	_____
service average	_____
# units transfused	_____
% of blood use	_____
# transfusion reviews	_____
# questionable	_____
# inappropriate	_____

NOSOCOMIAL INFECTION REVIEW

# patients with nosocomial infections	___/___%
TYPE: clean surgical wounds	___/___%
sepsis from central line	___/___%
pulmonary	___/___%
urinary	___/___%
other: list	___/___%
	___/___%
	___/___%

PHARMACY AND THERAPEUTICS

# patients reviewed for drug utilization	_____
# questionable	___/___%
# inappropriate	___/___%
# interventions by pharmacy	
re: ordering	_____
# service average	_____

MORBIDITY AND MORTALITY

Average severity index of patients	_____
service average	_____
# cardiac/respiratory arrest	_____
# questionable management	___/___%
# inappropriate management	___/___%
# deaths	_____
# questionable management	___/___%
# inappropriate management	___/___%

UTILIZATION REVIEW

# admission denials	_____
PRO	_____
Internal	_____
# denials repealed	_____
Average LOS	_____
service average	_____
# unnecessary days prior to surgery	_____
# inappropriate resource utilization	_____
# inappropriate special care utilization	_____

MEDICAL RECORD REVIEW

Delinquent Records	_____
service average	_____
# days suspended	_____
report to BMQA	_____
# reviewed for clinical pertinence	_____
# appropriate	_____
# documentation inappropriate	_____
Timeliness problems	_____
Legibility problems	_____
Other _____	

Reviewed by: _____ Date: _____
(Dept/Service Chief)

(continued)

QRM Summary for Reappointment (continued)

MEDICAL STAFF REAPPOINTMENT PROFILE

CURRENT STATUS:

Name: _____ Status: _____

Department/Service: _____

Specialty: _____ Subspecialty: _____

On file: License _____ DEA _____

CME Activities (hours): Internal _____ External _____

Department and Committee Meeting Attendance:

Title of Group	Dates	Attended	Excused	Unexcused
_____	_____	_____	_____	_____
_____	_____	_____	_____	_____
_____	_____	_____	_____	_____

QA/UM/RISK MANAGEMENT ISSUES

Date	Summary	Status/Resolution
_____	_____	_____
_____	_____	_____
_____	_____	_____

PROFESSIONAL LIABILITY CLAIMS

Summary	Date Settled	Settlement (list hospital costs separately)
_____	_____	_____
_____	_____	_____
_____	_____	_____

DISCIPLINARY ACTIONS

Date	Summary	Outcome
_____	_____	_____
_____	_____	_____
_____	_____	_____

HEALTH STATUS   no restrictions _____

Restrictions: _____
_____

Have there been any occurrences related to behavior, personality, or change in health status or judgment making?   Yes _____   No _____

Summary, if yes _____
_____
_____

(continued)

QRM Summary for Reappointment (continued)

DEPARTMENT CHAIRPERSON REVIEW

Date of review of QRM Summary: _____

Has the practitioner demonstrated competence in the privileges granted?

Granted privileges not performed within the previous two years:

Privileges performed outside granted privilege list:

Based on performance, should privileges be modified, reduced, withdrawn, expanded?

Yes _____ No _____

Recommendation	Reference Data from Profile
_____	_____
_____	_____
_____	_____
_____	_____
_____	_____

REAPPOINTMENT RECOMMENDATION

Based on the above review, the following is recommended:

Reappointment _____ Nonreappointment _____

Reason: _____
_____
_____

All Privileges Requested _____ Privileges Restricted _____

Reason: _____
_____
_____

Accept Resignation _____

Reason: _____
_____
_____

_____   _____

Department/Service Chief   Date

APPROVALS

_____   _____

Executive Committee Chairperson   Date

_____   _____

Board of Governors Chairperson   Date

FIGURE B.2. *Physician QA summary includes blanks for recording a physician's number and percentage of various types of adverse patient occurrences.*

SOURCE: *Medical staff reappointment profile.* Q Resource Monitor *(updates for Vol II) 5(5), Sept-Dec 1989. (adapted from MMAI composite and Kaiser Permanente, Los Angeles, QA Summary.)*

Quality Assurance Monitoring/Assessment for Reappointment to the Medical Staff

Reappointment   Assessment covering
_____ to _____   _____ to _____

Name of Practitioner

I. Departmental monitors
   A. Total number of patients/cases practitioner cared for during past year _____
   B. Number of practitioners' cases monitored _____
   C. Number of deficiencies _____
   D. Types of deficiencies _____
      _____
      _____
      _____
      _____

   E. Patterns/assessment of deficiencies

II. Surgical case review
   A. Total number of surgeries practitioner performed _____
   B. Number of these cases reviewed _____
   C. Number of deficiencies _____ Not applicable _____
   D. Patterns/assessment of deficiencies _____
      _____
      _____
      _____
      _____

III. Medical record review
   A. Number of practitioner's medical records performed _____
   B. Quality of record
      1. Number of deficiencies _____
      2. Nature of deficiencies _____
         _____
         _____
         _____
      3. Patterns/assessment of deficiencies—specify and describe
   C. Timeliness of dictation
      1. Number of times admitting privileges suspended or fines incurred
      2. Patterns/assessment of deficiencies
         _____ Total late H&Ps
         _____ Total late operative reports
         _____ Total late discharge summaries

IV. Drug usage
   A. Number of practitioner's patients for whom drug usage was monitored _____
   B. Problems recorded
      1. Number of adverse drug reactions _____
      2. Other _____
         _____
   C. Patterns/assessment of deficiencies
      _____ None
      _____ Specify and describe _____
         _____
         _____

(continued)

Quality Assurance Monitoring/Assessment for Reappointment to the Medical Staff (continued)

V. Blood and blood product monitors
   A. Number of practitioner's patients for whom blood and blood product usage was monitored
   B. Number of deficiencies
   C. Patterns/assessment
      _____ None
      _____ Specify and describe _____
      _____
      _____

VI. Utilization review
   A. Total number of PRO denials _____
      _____ Intensity/severity denials
      _____ Readmission within seven days denials
   B. Case mix problem patterns/assessment _____
      _____
      _____

VII. Incidents or problems reported by other professionals or administration:
   A. Number _____
   B. Patterns/assessment of deficiencies
      _____ None
      _____ Specify and describe _____
      _____
      _____

VIII. Malpractice claims
   A. Total number _____
   B. Patterns/assessment
      _____ None
      _____ Specify and describe _____
      _____
      _____

FIGURE B.3. *Physician QA profile asking for patterns of care discovered through monitoring and evaluation.*

QA Profile

NAME: _____ DEPARTMENT: _____

COMMITTEE ASSIGNMENTS: _____

FUNCTION	PERIOD COVERED			
	JAN-JUN (YR)	JUL-DEC (YR)	JAN-JUN (YR)	JUL-DEC (YR)

Volume Data
# Admissions 	
# Procedures 	
  - Inpatient
  - Ambulatory				

% Attendance
  - Dept meetings
  - Committee meetings
  - Medical staff meetings				

CME hours				
Performance Data				
Occurrence Screens				
Focused Reviews				
Surgical Case Review (ie, # of cases not meeting criteria/# cases reviewed)				
Transfusion Review (ie, # of cases not meeting criteria/# cases reviewed)				
Drug Usage Evaluation (ie, # of cases not meeting criteria/# cases reviewed)				
Medical Record Review (ie, # of charts not meeting criteria/# charts reviewed, medical care delinquency rate)				
Utilization Review (ie, DRG variations, LOS, etc)				
Risk Management (ie, # of claims, final settlements, patient complaints, compliments)				
Infection Control (Infection rates, nosocomial—surgical wound)				

MD Signature _____   _____   _____   _____

Dept Chairman Signature _____   _____   _____   _____

FIGURE B.4. *Physician QA profile with spaces for recording quarterly QA results.*
SOURCE: *Anne Arundel Medical Center, Annapolis, MD. Used with permission.*

Physician Quality Assurance

Custom Designed for DEMONSTRATION MEMORIAL HOSPITAL

INDIVIDUAL PHYSICIAN ANALYSIS & GRAPHING   © 1987 by AUTO-MED INC. : Omaha, Nebraska

1	2	3	4	5	6	7	8	9	10	11	12	13	14	15	16	17	18	19	20	21	22
MD ID NUMBER	SPECL'T NUMBER	TOTAL ADMITS	TOTAL CONSUL	TOTAL PROCDS	NORMAL TISSUE	MALPRC CLAIMS	SEYDEX NUMBER	C.M.E. HOURS	SG-TRF RATE	MORTAL RATE	RE-ADM RATE	PADMIT RATE	CONT'N DENIAL	ICU TR RATE	OPS TR DENIAL	INC'NT RATE	MON'G FAL'OT	SUSP'N RATE	NOSOCM RATE	CCMP'L RATE	DELAY START
1003	6	450	199*	400	4	4	9	5	%1	%6	%4	%3	%3	%33*	%2	%49*	%49*	%33	%24*	%21	%44

	3	4	5	6	7	8	9	10	11	12	13	14	15	16	17	18	19	20	21	22
>3 STD. DEV.																				
+3 STD. DEV.																				
+2 STD. DEV.																				
+1 STD. DEV.		X											X		X	X		X		
THE MEAN	X		X	X	X	X	X	X	X	X	X	X		X			X		X	X
−1 STD. DEV.																				
−2 STD. DEV.																				
−3 STD. DEV.																				
<3 STD. DEV.																				
MONITOR # →	3	4	5	6	7	8	9	10	11	12	13	14	15	16	17	18	19	20	21	22
MEAN →	332	78	214	9	4	9	4	2	6	4	4	5	11	5	16	20	26	9	22	25
Std Dev →	183	80	186	6	2	7	2	2	4	1	3	5	13	3	19	17	27	10	8	20

* = +/− one standard deviation   ** = +/− two standard deviations   *** = +/− three standard deviations

FIGURE B.5. *Display of physician-specific indicator data. Statistical analysis shows how close the physician is to the medical staff mean for each indicator.*
SOURCE: *Freed R, Adwers J: Tracking quality assurance activity: A PC-based computerized system.* QA and Utilization Review 3(4):109, Nov 1988.

Cross-Monitoring Provider Profile*

Provider Physician 95	Monitoring Completed Between 7/1/75 And 7/1/76	Number of Monitoring Periods 3	Total Number of Records Monitored 20	Total Deficiencies Attributed to the Provider 9

Indicator Class and Type \ Def. Cause	DOC	Knowl. Skill	Knew, Didn't Do	Lack Equip	Lack Pers	Policy, Proc.	M.R. Forms	Over-util	Environ-mental	Other	Total
JUSTIFICATION Diagnosis, Problem			1								1
Surgery											
Procedure											
Admission											
OUTCOME Discharge Status	5										5
Pt Knowledge											
Follow-up Plan											
Mortality			1								1
INDICATOR Length of Time								2			2
Critical Process											
Critical Clue											
Comp/Crit. Mgt.											
TOTAL	5		2					2			9

*Complete one profile for each provider audited during period

FIGURE B.6. *A completed profile for one physician monitored during a 12-month period. Indicator occurrences are grouped by type of cause.*
SOURCE: *Adapted from Fox L, Stearns G, Imbiorski W:* The Masters Manual for the Advanced Training of Hospital Audit Specialists, *Chicago: Care Communications, 1977, p 189.*

Reappointment Summary Form and Recommendation

Physician: *Art Throscopy*   First Appointed to Staff: *1980*   Dept.: *Orthopedics*   Age: *42*
Staff Category: *Active*   ☐ If different from current category, check here and explain under Comments.

SUMMARY OF PERFORMANCE EVALUATION BY DEPARTMENT CHAIRMAN*

The physician's performance has been reviewed by his/her Department Chairman and found satisfactory in the following areas:

	YES	NO	QUALIFIED ANSWER
1. Current state license and controlled substance registrations.	✔		
2. Current liability insurance in adequate amount.	✔		
3. No liability claims filed or settled since last reappointment.	✔		
4. Sufficient activity at the hospital to allow review of clinical competence.	✔		
5. Sufficient activity to maintain proficiency for requested privileges.	✔		
6. Satisfactory performance as demonstrated by review of information from quality assurance/risk management and medical staff peer review monitors.	✔		
7. No more than one suspension for delinquent medical records.		✔	
8. Satisfactory participation in required medical staff functions.			✔
9. Good working relationships with others.			✔
10. Satisfactory performance in all other hospitals and health facilities since last reappointment.	✔		
11. No adverse actions recorded in state, federal, or other data banks.	✔		
12. Privileges recommended are the same as requested.	✔		
13. Continuing medical education requirements met.	✔		

*All "no" and "qualified answers" must be explained under Comments.

Comments: *Dr. Throscopy was counseled concerning behavior. No problems have recurred. He also has been counseled concerning record completion and meeting attendance.*

RECOMMENDATION OF MEDICAL EXECUTIVE COMMITTEE

_____ The physician meets all requirements for demonstrating current clinical competence, ability to work with others, and compliance with bylaws, rules, and regulations. Reappointment and renewal of privileges as requested is recommended.

_✔_ The physician meets requirements for current clinical competence and should be reappointed and granted privileges as requested, but should receive a letter stating that improvement is needed in the following areas:

_✔_ Timely medical record completion   _✔_ Participation in medical staff affairs
_✔_ Ability to work with others   _____ Issues raised in quality assurance or peer review
_____ Other: _____
_____ The physician should be reappointed with the following modifications or limitations on the privileges requested: _____
_____ The physician should not be reappointed because of the failure to resolve concerns over:
_____ Current clinical competence   _____ Ability to work with others
_____ Failure to comply with bylaws, rules, and regulations   _____ Other: _____
☐ If the above recommendation of the MEC differs from that of either the Department Chairman or Credentials Committee, check here and explain. _____

Signed: *Sherman T. Potter, MD,* Chairman, Medical Executive Committee

FIGURE B.7. *Reappointment summary and recommendation form summarizes examination of the physician's QA results and asks for a final decision on reappointment.*
SOURCE: *Quality agenda: Reappointment of Dr. Art Throscopy.* Quality Letter 1(5):17, Dec 1989-Jan 1990.

Sample Format for Board Quality of Care Committee Review of a Recommendation for Physician Reappointment

Name _____ Dr 005 _____   Dept/Specialty ____ Obstetrics ____   Age ___ 41 ___

Element   ASSESSMENT
_____

Activity: No problems

200 admissions
 30 consultations
134 deliveries

QA Reviews: All cases met standard of care

All cases reviewed,
19 cases sent to peer review

Malpractice Cases/Adverse Actions: Department chief reviewed records in all 3
3 new cases filed since last reappointment   cases, including plantiff's filings. Finds no
                                                       negligence in any.

Behavioral Issues:

2 incidents reported; serious   Physician apologized to nurse; resident was
disagreement with nurse and resident.   found at fault and disciplined; no behavioral
                                                       concerns.

Recommendation:

I find this physician fully qualified and recommend reappointment without reservation.

                                                       Jack Jones
                                                       Chief, OB/GYN

Figure B.8. Form allows the governing body to look at QA findings in preparation for making a decision on a physician's reappointment.
Source: Sample formats for board oversight of QA and credentialing. Q Resource Monitor *special supplement*, 4(1):9, Jan-Feb 1988.

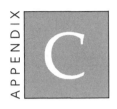

APPENDIX

How to Use Control Charts to Set Thresholds for Evaluation and Track Indicator Data Against Them

In cases where guidance is needed as to when a data pattern should trigger further investigation, applying thresholds becomes useful. *An indicator data threshold is the point at which a stimulus (eg, a single rate or pattern in rates) is strong enough to signal the need for response and the beginning of the process of determining why the threshold has been crossed.* The upward trend in data depicted in Figure C.1. and the isolated elevations in Figure C.2. are patterns that may be strong enough to trigger further investigation. These patterns may serve as thresholds.

Numerical levels as thresholds

A predetermined numerical level may be used as a threshold, meaning that further evaluation must occur when this numerical level is crossed. The control chart is well suited for application of numerical thresholds. There the threshold is plotted directly onto the graph in the form of control or specification limit lines. When a measurement crosses the control limit lines, as do the two isolated elevated measurements in Figure C.3., further investigation must occur.

The numerical level that serves as the threshold for sentinel event indicators is zero. A sentinel event occurrence, by definition, is serious every time it occurs (eg, a preventable trauma death due to undetected and untreated tension pneumothorax). Therefore, 100% of sentinel event occurrences must be reviewed. Figure C.4. depicts the threshold for all sentinel event indicators.

Setting numerical levels that serve as thresholds for rate-based indicators is more complex. Currently, there are three ways to determine such levels: expert consensus, definition of internal organizational objectives, and calculating a derived range around a statistical mean (calculated from data collected and adjusted, when necessary, for case mix).

The latter approach to determining numerical levels that will serve as thresholds for rate-based indicators involves statistics and requires a data base that will progressively accumulate data and calculate the statistical mean and a range around that mean.

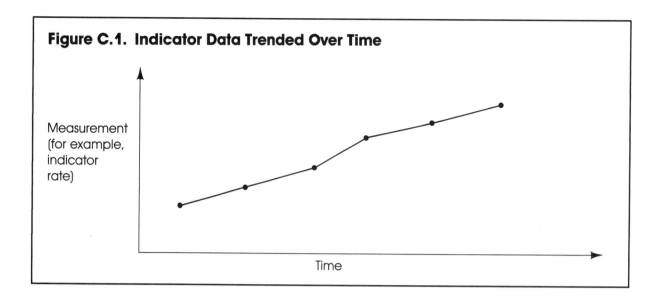

Figure C.1. Indicator Data Trended Over Time

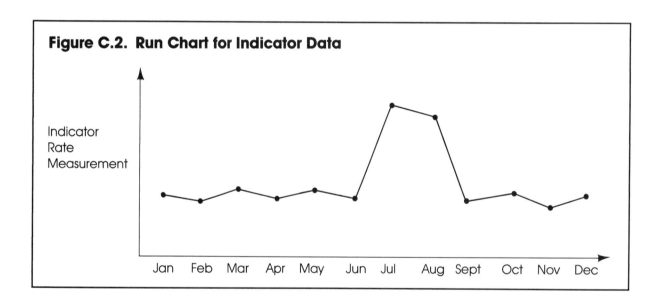

Figure C.2. Run Chart for Indicator Data

Individual hospitals or departments may establish their own data base, using internal data collected continuously. Alternately, a number of hospitals may pool their indicator data to obtain group-specific and organization-specific information that can be used to improve the quality of care internally by each participating hospital.

The derivation of statistical thresholds and their use as control limits is discussed in the following text. This approach to setting numerical thresholds involves calculating the mean and the standard deviation of the mean for a data distribution and then setting the threshold at one, two, or three times the standard deviation.

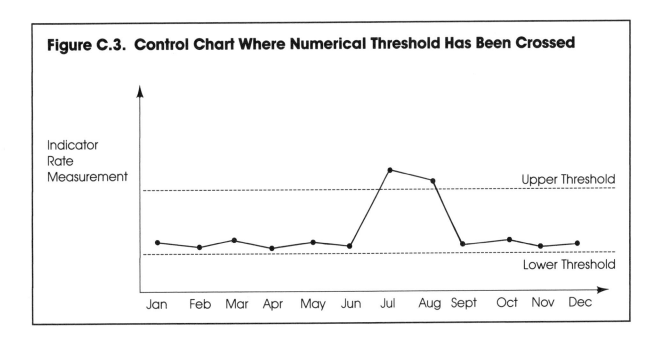

Figure C.3. Control Chart Where Numerical Threshold Has Been Crossed

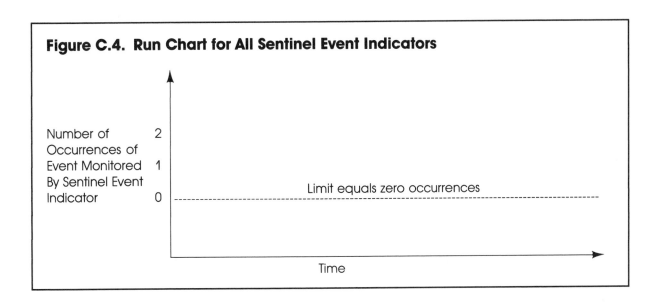

Figure C.4. Run Chart for All Sentinel Event Indicators

Using numbers to describe data: Calculating the mean

Numerical descriptions of a data set provide additional information that is useful in evaluating data. Two commonly used numerical descriptions of a data distribution are measures of central tendency and measures of variability.

A measure of central tendency is a number that locates the approximate center of a distribution of data. One of the best understood measures of central location is the mean or average of a data set. The mean is the sum of all the measurements divided by the total number of measurements in the data set (see Figure C.5.).

The mean can be charted directly onto a run chart (see Figure C.6.), a control chart, and/or other types of graphs.

What can the mean of a data set tell users? The mean is useful in determining baseline rates for monitored processes and outcomes and in providing a reference point for organizations interested in continuously improving the quality of care relative to an indicator-monitored process or outcome.

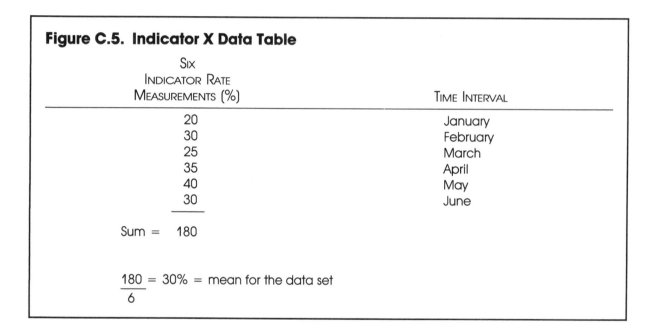

Figure C.5. Indicator X Data Table

SIX INDICATOR RATE MEASUREMENTS (%)	TIME INTERVAL
20	January
30	February
25	March
35	April
40	May
30	June

Sum =   180

$\frac{180}{6}$ = 30% = mean for the data set

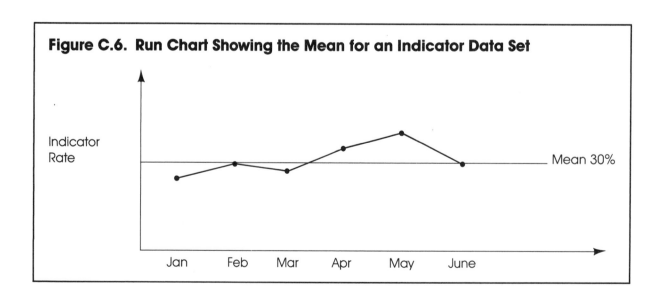

Figure C.6. Run Chart Showing the Mean for an Indicator Data Set

Indicator Rate

Mean 30%

Jan   Feb   Mar   Apr   May   June

In the early stages of indicator use by organizations, the mean for an indicator data set can be used to determine the baseline or "usual" rate for the occurrence of the event monitored by an indicator. For many key processes and outcomes monitored by indicators, these baselines are not yet known. This information is important because without it, organizations cannot measure improvement, deterioration, or steadiness in the quality, of patient care they provide, relative to a monitored process or outcome.

Measuring variability: Standard deviation

One limitation of the mean is that it does not provide a descriptive measure of the variability of indicator rate measurements relative to their mean. This is important information because indicator rate measurements that demonstrate a high degree of variability suggest that there may be important quality-of-care questions that should be asked.

To complete the description of a data set requires a *measure of its variability*, that is, a number that describes the spread or variation in the distribution of the data. One common measure of the variability of a data distribution is the standard deviation. A large standard deviation relative to the mean shows that the rates are widely spread out from their mean. This suggests that there is a large degree of variability relative to the event that the indicator is monitoring. A small standard deviation relative to the mean shows that the rates are closely concentrated around their mean. This suggests that there is little variability relative to the event the indicator is monitoring.

A normal distribution enables one to observe where individual measurements (for example, indicator rates) lie—in terms of multiples of the standard deviation—within a given distance from the mean. In theory, one can calculate for a normal distribution the proportion of rates that lie within one, two, and three times the standard deviation of the mean. In a normal distribution, only 1 in 20 rates will differ from the mean by more than twice the standard deviation.

Two standard deviations may be used as control limits for indicator data. These control limits, when crossed, are intended to stimulate organizations to further investigate the event that the indicator is monitoring (ie, the control limits are thresholds for evaluation).

Calculation of the standard deviation for a short series of figures, such as monthly indicator rates, involves five steps. Consider that the monthly rate measurements for indicator X are 29%, 30%, 34%, 40%, 28%, and 26%, as listed below. First, each of these individual numbers are squared and the sum of these squares calculated (a).

Six Indicator Rate Measurements	Square of Each Rate Measurement
29	841
30	900
34	1156
40	1600
28	784
26	676
Sum 187	5957 = a

Second, the sum of the measurements (187) is squared and divided by the total number of measurements (in this series there are 6 indicator rate measurements):

$$187 \times 187 = 34969$$

$$\frac{34969}{6} = 5828 = b$$

Third, b is subtracted from a:

$$5957 - 5828 = 129$$

This gives the sum of the squared deviations of the measurements around their own mean. Fourth, this value (ie, 129) is divided by $n-1$ to reach the variance; n is the number of measurements (ie, 6):

$$\frac{129}{5} = 26 \text{ (variance)}$$

Fifth, the square root of the variance (that is, 26) is taken to reach the standard deviation:

$$\sqrt{26} = 5 \text{ (standard deviation)}$$

For the data set presented above, two standard deviations relative to the mean of 31 would be: 31 plus or minus 10, that is, 41 and 21, respectively. Therefore, only one in 20 rate measurements would be expected to be below 21 or above 41 (ie, differ from the mean by more than twice its standard deviation).

CONTROL CHARTS

These measurements may be plotted onto a run chart. A run chart that has a measurement of the historic variability plotted on the chart is called a *control chart*; the plotted measure of variability is called a *control limit*. Control limits are often set at one, two, or three times the standard deviation of the mean for the data set (Figure C.7.). The control limits can be used as thresholds for evaluation; in that case, when data breaches the control limits, the organization must evaluate the related care and services to see if an opportunity to improve exists.

When a measurement crosses a control limit, the reasons are unclear until further investigation occurs. This point bears emphasis. There may be a tendency to assume that if rates are within the expected range (ie, do not cross control limits), care is of expected and therefore acceptable quality. Conversely, when rates cross control limits there is a tendency to assume that care is of unexpected and therefore unacceptable quality. These assumptions, however, may be erroneous.

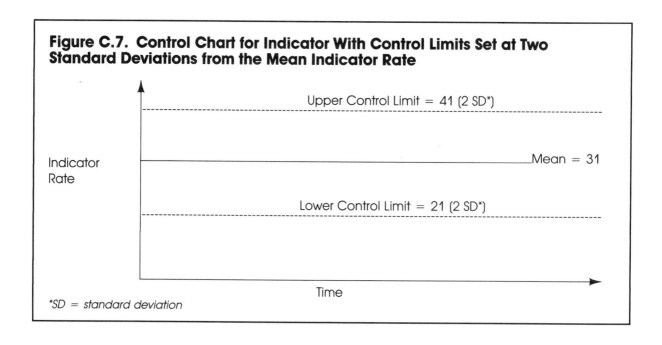

Figure C.7. Control Chart for Indicator With Control Limits Set at Two Standard Deviations from the Mean Indicator Rate

Indicator Rate

Upper Control Limit = 41 (2 SD*)

Mean = 31

Lower Control Limit = 21 (2 SD*)

Time

*SD = standard deviation

The statistical mean identifies the "usual" or statistically normative value and may not necessarily represent the most desirable value. For example, consider that the statistical mean for patients' length of stay in 100 emergency departments is some lengthy amount of time. This normative value probably does not represent the most desirable value, which, according to patients, their families, and many others, should be lower. Hospital emergency department #1, therefore, whose rate happens to fall outside control limits for the indicator data set (eg, greater than two standard deviations *below* the mean) may actually be providing better care relative to the monitored event than hospital emergency department #2 whose rate lies within the expected range (eg, within two standard deviations of the mean). Conversely, hospital emergency department #2 whose rate lies within the expected range may actually be providing care that can and should be improved.

Further, the usefulness of statistical means and control limits depend on the reliability and validity of indicators and the data they generate. Considerable effort must be devoted to ensuring that indicators are reliable and valid measures of performance because of the wide range of activities potentially triggered within organizations by statistical information derived from indicator data. The potential for human fallibility warrants caution by those who evaluate and use data, especially during the early stages of performance monitoring and evaluation.

In summary

Organizing and describing indicator data through use of graphs and numerical descriptions increase the probability that users can focus attention on important aspects of data and draw conclusions. This is the goal of a threshold for evaluation: to focus attention (ie, in-depth evaluation) on findings that one has reason to believe indicate a significant opportunity to improve (eg, an opportunity to reduce variations in outcomes). Important numerical descriptions of a data distribution include the mean and standard deviation. The mean is a measure of central tendency of a data distribution. The standard deviation is a measure of the variability of a data distribution relative to its mean.